D1546306

BORDERLINE PATIENTS

BORDERLINE PATIENTS

*Extending the Limits
of Treatability*

HAROLD W. KOENIGSBERG, M.D.

OTTO F. KERNBERG, M.D.

MICHAEL H. STONE, M.D.

ANN H. APPELBAUM, M.D.

FRANK E. YEOMANS, M.D.

DIANA DIAMOND, PH.D.

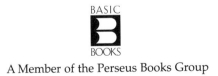

BASIC
BOOKS

A Member of the Perseus Books Group

A CIP catalog record for this book is available from the Library of Congress.
ISBN 0-465-09560-7

FIRST EDITION

00 01 02 03 / 10 9 8 7 6 5 4 3 2 1

Contents

Preface

The goal of this book, which builds on our previous work on the treatment of borderline patients, is to delineate an approach for some of the more difficult situations encountered by therapists who work with these patients. It is an outgrowth of our systematic articulation of a psychodynamic psychotherapy for borderline patients, an approach that derives from an ego psychology and object relations model. We have identified the sources of a number of impediments that arise all too often: an inability to establish more than a tenuous treatment relationship in the first place; entrenched interpersonal patterns that surface once treatment is under way; the complicating effect of common comorbid conditions such as depression. It is our hope that some of the perspectives and tactics we present here can broaden the range of borderline patients who benefit from treatment.

We codified the principles and practice of transference-focused psychotherapy (TFP)—a form of psychodynamic psychotherapy tailored to the treatment of borderline patients—in our first work, *Psychodynamic Psychotherapy of Borderline Patients* (Kernberg, Selzer, Koenigsberg, Carr, and Appelbaum 1989), and developed them further in a work informed by the study of recorded research cases as part of a National Institute of Mental Health (NIMH) treatment development grant, *Psychotherapy for Borderline Personality* (Clarkin, Yeomans, and Kernberg 1999). We have also described in detail the contract-setting phase of TFP, in *Treating the Borderline Patient* (Yeomans, Selzer, and Clarkin 1992). We have always sought to strike a balance between an operationalized description of treatment that could be communicated in the most clinically accessible fashion (and the most uniform for research purposes) and an approach that does justice to the individual differences among patients, to their individual defensive and coping styles, and to the diversity of emotionally pressing concerns each patient brings to each hour.

All of the books cited here introduce the fundamentals of TFP, which was designed for application to the more severe *DSM-IV* Axis II personality disorders (borderline, histrionic, narcissistic, paranoid, schizoid, and schizotypal) and to some, not otherwise specified, that are structured at the borderline level of organization (a construct reviewed in chapters 1 and 2). This book presumes that the reader is familiar with psychodynamic treatment and offers an overview of TFP in the first chapter.

The next two chapters provide two different vantage points from which to think about patients who respond slowly or not at all to TFP. Chapter 2 sketches in broad strokes the complex interaction between biological endowment, early (infant-caregiver) relationships, and unfolding life events. Although much of the basic science of personality development has yet to be translated into methods for the consulting room, the chapter alerts the clinician to the potential role of ancillary biological interventions and to the impact of attachment patterns and the corresponding usefulness of attending to them. Chapter 3 revisits the conventional wisdom that accurate diagnosis is a sine qua non for treatment. This reassessment is especially relevant because so many dramatic presentations of other disorders are mistaken for borderline personality disorder (BPD); these patients, who are not expected to respond to TFP, account for some of the "difficult" cases.

The seven chapters constituting part 2, the core of the book, address the complicating factors in the treatment of borderline personality patients that occur with relative frequency: particular personality patterns, histories of traumatic experiences in childhood, problematic attachment styles, erotic transferences and countertransferences, and comorbid depressions. The final part discusses the use of such complementary resources as dream analysis, pharmacotherapy, and the sequential adoption of different modalities to extend the reach of effective treatment for borderline patients.

This work took shape at the Personality Disorder Institute at the New York Presbyterian Hospital, Westchester Division, directed by Otto Kernberg and codirected by John Clarkin, and before that in the Borderline Psychotherapy Research Project, led by John Clarkin and Harold Koenigsberg at the New York Hospital—Cornell Medical Center. The authors wish to express their thanks to John Clarkin, a vital contributor to the research program, whose vision, judgment, and scientific sophistication have been invaluable. We thank our colleagues at the Personality Disorder Institute: Drs. Steven Bauer, Arthur Carr, Pamela Foelsch, Catherine Haran, Paulina Kernberg, Sonia Kulchcky, and Lawrence Rockland, who have conducted recorded psychotherapies and supervised therapists as part of the systematic study, and who have contributed their clinical and theoretical wisdom. They are friends as well as colleagues.

Those who made important contributions to the ideas in this book include Drs. John Clarkin, Pamela Foelsch, Hilary Levine, and Kenneth Levy, on attachment, and Dr. Thomas Smith, on better conceptualizations of paranoid regressions. Help with the chapters on trauma, countertransference, and sequential treatment was provided by Drs. Judit Gordon-Lendvay, Eric Fertuck, and William Deal in the form of literature searches, advice, and case material. We also thank Drs. Mary Main and Erik Hesse, whose critical reading of the chapter on attachment status improved it immeasurably, and the many postdoctoral fellows, residents, and scholars who have visited and trained in our institute. We have benefited from their wisdom and expertise. Portions of chapter 12 appeared in Harold W. Koenigsberg, "Integrating Psychotherapy and Pharmacotherapy in Treating Borderline Patients," in *In Session: Psychotherapy in Practice* (John Wiley & Sons, Inc., 1997, vol. 3, pp. 39–56).

We are grateful to our department chairmen, Drs. Robert Michels and Jack Barchas, who have encouraged our work, each in his own way—Dr. Michels by consulting substantively with us on an ongoing basis, always offering a rich perspective, and Dr. Barchas by fostering both our research and clinical endeavors. The first author, now at the Mount Sinai School of Medicine, thanks Dr. Kenneth Davis for his encouragement and support. We would also like to thank our editor at Basic Books, Cindy Hyden, without whose efforts this book would not have come to fruition.

Harold W. Koenigsberg
Otto F. Kernberg
Michael H. Stone
Ann H. Appelbaum
Frank E. Yeomans
Diana Diamond

NEW YORK CITY AND
WHITE PLAINS, NEW YORK

PART ONE
REVISITING THE
FUNDAMENTALS

CHAPTER 1

Borderline Patients and Transference-Focused Psychotherapy

Borderline patients have acquired a reputation as "difficult" patients, and the diagnosis has taken on a pejorative connotation. This is unfortunate because, in our view, borderline patients can often be helped enormously. Their many strengths are often overlooked in the Sturm und Drang of their dramatic and turbulent symptomatology. In conflict-free areas, their intellectual faculties are impressive. Borderline patients are often articulate and closely attuned to their surroundings; their interpersonal sensitivity presents as a liability early on, but it can turn into a valuable asset later in life.

By no means atypical is the course of Mrs. R., now a fifty-five-year-old Hispanic woman who first tried to kill herself in college, made several more serious attempts in the succeeding years, and was arrested in her early twenties for threatening her boyfriend with a gun. She had been hospitalized many times, including one stay of almost a year, and had been in treatment with four different therapists. On discharge from her final hospitalization, a senior consultant told her that unless she could become genuinely engaged in therapy, she would probably either kill herself or end up in jail. Perhaps chastened by this dire prognosis, and possibly through the grace of a fortunate referral and her own personal strengths, she was able to engage in a ten-year course of psychotherapy. Over this time, her self-destructiveness ended, she married a caring and reliable man, and she gave birth to three children. She developed her own business, which flourished, and she was able to enjoy the roles of wife and mother as well. At the age of fifty-five, however, she presented again for psychiatric treatment, following a financial setback in her business that had precipitated symptoms of a mild episode of major depressive disorder. She rapidly responded to antidepressant treatment and reported that, in dealing with this depression, she made use of what she had learned in psychotherapy to stay grounded as she dealt with the setback.

Nevertheless, we do not want to minimize the challenge that borderline patients present; many do not have the fortunate outcome of Mrs. R. The prognosis is often guarded. About 10 percent of borderline patients die by suicide. A number of treatment approaches have been developed, including modified psychodynamic psychotherapy, supportive psychotherapy (Rockland 1992), forms of cognitive-behavioral therapy, including dialectic-behavior therapy (DBT) (Linehan 1993), and the use of a variety of medications. Empirical data supporting each of these modalities are now available (Perry et al. 1999). What is less clear is whether some patients respond better to one modality rather than another, and whether different modalities foster different types of change. For example, medication may reduce impulsivity and affective instability, DBT may mitigate the misery and interpersonal consequences of affective instability, and psychodynamic psychotherapy may foster a more integrated sense of identity and a more realistic view of others.

We and our colleagues at the Personality Disorder Institute of the Weill Medical School of Cornell University and the New York Presbyterian Hospital have been studying the diagnosis and treatment of patients with borderline personality disorders over the last two decades. During this time, we refined a form of psychodynamic psychotherapy adapted for borderline patients—transference-focused psychotherapy (TFP). The treatment emphasizes use of the transference to surface and vividly present to patients the principal internalized object relations that shape their relationships to self and others. We have studied this method in recorded psychotherapy sessions (with the patient's informed consent) conducted by senior clinicians, taught it to psychotherapists outside of our group, and trained psychiatric residents and psychology interns in its use. We describe the approach in *Psychodynamic Psychotherapy of Borderline Patients* (Kernberg, Selzer, Koenigsberg, Appelbaum, and Carr 1989) and developed it further in the form of a treatment manual, *Psychotherapy for Borderline Personality* (Clarkin, Yeomans, and Kernberg 1999).

In the course of our work, we have encountered borderline patients who posed special challenges to treatment. Some of these patients were unusually difficult to engage in treatment in the first place. Others initially appeared to use psychotherapy effectively, then entered into interminable treatment stalemates. Some either developed regressions of psychotic proportions or escalated dangerous acting-out behavior; some just dropped out of treatment precipitously. Our experience seems to parallel that of colleagues who have seen borderline patients repeatedly fail after trials of treatment in a variety of modalities, carried out by experienced clinicians. Although we do not presuppose that all borderline patients can be helped at all points in their lives, we have attempted to adapt our psychodynamic approach to better engage those who are particularly resistant to treatment. Some patients may benefit from an integrated approach—treatment with two or more modalities concurrently. For others, being treated first with a single modality may be prerequisite to more ambitious work later on.

This volume focuses on work with the particularly challenging borderline patient. It draws on our own work in the Personality Disorder Institute and before that in the Borderline Research Group at the Westchester Division of the New York Hospital–Cornell Medical Center. We examine the factors that limit the treatability of borderline patients with transference-focused psychotherapy and explore approaches for extending these limits. We begin by reviewing the concept of borderline personality organization and present an object relations model of its intrapsychic structure. Using this framework, we review the basic methods of transference-focused psychotherapy.

BORDERLINE PERSONALITY ORGANIZATION

Transference-focused psychotherapy is rooted in the conceptually based and clinically useful construct of borderline personality *organization* (BPO) developed by Otto Kernberg (1967)—as distinguished from the symptom- and behavior-based diagnosis identified by *DSM-IV* for borderline personality *disorder* (BPD) (see figure 1-1). According to Kernberg's construct of BPO, a borderline individual is characterized by:

FIGURE 1-1   *DSM=IV* Diagnostic Criteria for Borderline Personality Disorder

A pervasive pattern of instability of interpersonal relationships, self-image, and affects marked by impulsivity beginning by early adulthood and present in a variety of contexts, as indicted by five (or more) of the following criteria:

1. Frantic efforts to avoid real or imagined abandonment. Note: Do not include suicidal or self-mutilating behavior covered in criterion 5.
2. A pattern of unstable and intense interpersonal relationships characterized by alternating between extremes of idealization and devaluation.
3. Identity disturbance: markedly and persistently unstable self-image or sense of self.
4. Impulsivity in at least two areas that are potentially self-damaging, such as spending, sex, substance abuse, reckless driving, binge eating. Note: Do not include suicidal or self-mutilating covered in criterion 5.
5. Recurrent suicidal behavior, gestures, or threats, or self-mutilating behavior.
6. Affective instability due to a marked reactivity of mood (for example, intense episodic dysphoria, irritability, or anxiety usually lasting a few hours and only rarely more than a few days).
7. Chronic feelings of emptiness.
8. Inappropriate intense anger or difficulty controlling anger (for example, frequent displays of temper, constant anger, recurrent physical fights).
9. Transient, stress-related, paranoid ideation or severe dissociative symptoms.

SOURCE: American Psychiatric Association: *Diagnostic and Statistical Manual of Mental Disorders*, 4th ed. (Washington, D.C.: American Psychiatric Association, 1994), p. 654.

- Primitive defense mechanisms
- Identity diffusion
- Generally intact reality testing

Primitive defenses and identity diffusion differentiate individuals with borderline organization from those with a neurotic personality organization. Generally intact reality testing differentiates them from psychotic individuals.

The BPO concept encompasses many of the personality disorders described as separate diagnoses in *DSM-IV* (narcissistic, histrionic, antisocial, paranoid, schizoid, and BPD). It is clinically useful because it describes a *range* of psychological functioning, which can be understood in terms of the object relations model that follows and can be treated with the methods of TFP, the psychodynamically oriented psychotherapy geared to working with patients with BPO.

The Object Relations Model of BPO

Defense mechanisms are the means developed by the mind to negotiate the conflicts that arise from the pressures exerted on the psyche by libidinal forces, aggressive forces, internalized prohibitions, and external reality. The individual whose psychological development proceeds successfully develops mature defense mechanisms (for example, intellectualization, humor, sublimation) that are nuanced and also flexible enough that the individual can adapt to the complexities of external reality as well as to internal psychological pressures. *Primitive* defense mechanisms are the developing infant's first psychological attempts to deal with the stress of conflicting forces; when psychological maturation is impeded, primitive defenses continue to function in the adult. These mechanisms are crude and rigid; they alleviate an individual's anxiety to some degree, but at the cost of going through life with a brittle and inflexible way of experiencing self and others.

The most fundamental primitive defense mechanism is *splitting,* which is at the root of borderline personality. An understanding of object relations theory is a precondition to understanding splitting, borderline personality organization, and the workings of TFP.

Libidinal and aggressive drives are fundamental to a psychoanalytic understanding of psychopathology. Object relations theory stresses the concept that drives should be considered in relation to the *object* of the drive. The basic "building block" of psychic structure is thus represented by a dyad involving a self representation and an object representation, linked by a particular affect (see figure 1-2a).

In the early stages of life, before object constancy is achieved—or, for that matter, self constancy—the developing being perceives different subjective states involving different experiences with others as totally separate and distinct from one another. So, for example, the experience of the hungry infant who is immediately satisfied by the available mother registers differently in the psyche from that of the same hungry infant when the mother, for whatever reason, is not available (see figures 1-2b and 1-2c). In the early stages of development, a single primary caregiver is experienced by the infant as two different others, each an exaggerated, unidimensional character: the all-good nurturer and the withholding depriver. These primitive representations of others correspond to the way borderline patients often experience and describe others.

FIGURE 1-2   The Object-Relation Dyad

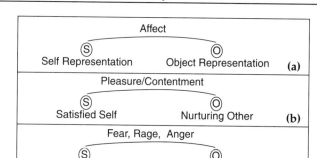

In successful psychological development, the individual integrates the different extremes into a complex, nuanced representation of the other—a realistic mix of good and bad (satisfying and frustrating) traits. With such integrated internal images in mind, the individual is prepared to deal with the complexities of the world. In other words, the individual's internal world corresponds relatively well to external reality.

In the case of borderline individuals, the integration of the early, separate, and extreme representations does not take place. As figure 1-3 demonstrates, their internal world remains divided as a result of the splitting defense.[1] Dyadic representations of opposite valence coexist side by side, inconsistent with each other, yet each with the potential to determine the individual's behavior in the moment.

It is this fragmented inner world that prevents the establishment of a unified sense of the individual's own identity and those of others. This is the *identity diffusion* cited by Kernberg as one of the three defining features of borderline organization. It can lead to a subjective sense of confusion about life goals, values, and sexual object choice, as well as a pervasive sense of boredom or emptiness. An individual whose internal world is so structured perceives the external world accordingly—in abrupt extremes. This perception explains many of the symptoms of borderline pathology: the rapidly shifting moods, the intense anger, the lack of a clear, stable sense of self, the

---

[1]See Clarkin, Yeomans, and Kernberg (1999) on why some internal worlds do not become integrated.

FIGURE 1-3   **The Split in Borderline Personality Disorder**

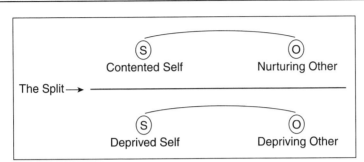

fear of abandonment (because there is no internal sense of a consistent, permanent other), the unstable and intense interpersonal relationships.

One might ask: How can this primitive system, which is so poorly adapted to reality, be considered a defense? It functions as a defense in that it protects the "good object" from the aggression and rage directed at the "bad object," so that in good moments the individual can maintain the sense of a perfect other who is able to satisfy all of her needs (idealization). The internal split in the psyche sustains the possibility of the perfect other, whereas psychological maturation, as represented by the integration of these extreme representations, actually entails a loss—of the imagined perfect other to the reality of the mix of good with bad. That loss corresponds to what Melanie Klein (1957) described as the "depressive position," echoing the need to mourn the longed-for ideal other, who in the early stages of life was felt to be real.

THE BASIC METHODS OF
TRANSFERENCE-FOCUSED PSYCHOTHERAPY

Transference-focused psychotherapy derives from the belief that individuals experience external reality through the structure of their inner world of internalized object relations dyads. This is particularly significant in the therapeutic situation because the patient lives out, *in the transference,* his predominant object relations dyads—experiencing the therapist as the corresponding other (see figures 1-4 and 1-5).

At any point in time, a particular object relations dyad is active in the transference. The work of TFP is based on identifying the patient's primary

FIGURE 1-4   The Borderline Patient's Internal World

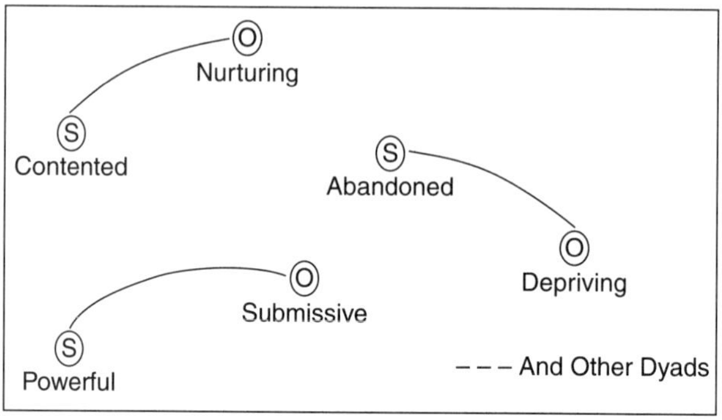

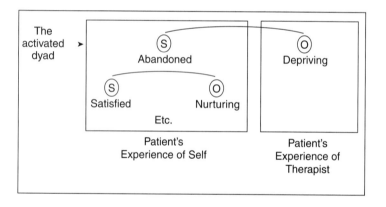

FIGURE 1-5   The Borderline Patient's Experience of the Therapist at a Given Moment

internal self and object representations as they occur in the therapeutic setting so that he or she, on achieving conscious awareness of them and of the reasons for them, will be able to integrate them into more complex internal representations, with the help of the therapist. The work is difficult because the therapist must largely infer these internal representations from the patient's behavior, and because the targeted awareness is painful and dangerous insofar as it threatens to destroy the precarious homeostasis that protects the image of the ideal other.

The TFP therapist must be alert to three channels of communication: the patient's verbal messages, his nonverbal messages, and the therapist's own countertransference. In the early stages of treatment, the most important in-formation is often obtained from the second and third channels; the patient's statements tend to stick to what he is already aware of, and the therapist is challenged to look beyond that.

The therapist must also be alert to the dynamics of object relations dyads as they play out in the transference.

Projections.   Borderline patients often attribute to the therapist a part of the object relations dyad that they cannot accept as being a part of their own makeup. For example, it is often very difficult for borderline patients to see themselves in the role of the aggressor or persecutor since, on a con-scious level, they experience a hatred of the persecutor. Of course, much of a borderline patient's self-destructive behavior can be conceptualized as ei-ther enacting the persecutor role against herself, or attacking herself be-cause she senses an identification with the persecutor role and cannot tolerate it. Very typically, however, the transference is shaped by the bor-derline patient's attribution of the aggressor or persecutor role to the thera-pist. Although this is the mechanism of projection, the borderline patient often goes a step further and tries to provoke the therapist to treat her badly, thus creating, in the real relationship, a dynamic that makes her pro-jection appear true. This process is the hallmark of the borderline defense mechanism, *projective identification.*

Oscillations.   The two poles of an object relations dyad may abruptly switch (see figure 1-6). These shifts may take place without any awareness on the part of the patient and may be observable only in his behavior. Take the ex-ample of a patient whose therapist is about to leave on vacation. A dyad in which the patient experiences self as a powerless, helpless, abandoned child, and the therapist as an all-powerful, unencumbered parent, is activated. The patient speaks in a weak and childlike manner of how vulnerable and de-fenseless he feels with the therapist leaving. Then, out of the patient's con-scious awareness, the two poles of the dyad suddenly reverse. The patient identifies with the powerful self-sufficient parent and treats the therapist as the vulnerable one. Suddenly the patient becomes angry and commanding in the session, berating the therapist for leaving, perhaps even making veiled threats of suicide that cause the therapist to have actual feelings of fear and vulnerability. Here there has been an oscillation of the object rela-tions dyad. When such sudden shifts occur, they frequently leave both the

FIGURE 1-6   Oscillation in an Object-Relation Dyad

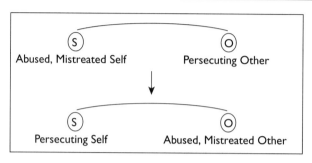

patient and the therapist confused and anxious. By staying alert to this phenomenon, however, the therapist can keep track of the dyads active in the patient's internal world.

Dyads Defending Against Other Dyads.   Another characteristic of the object relations dyads that the therapist must be attentive to is the way in which one dyad can defend against another. A typical example is seen in figure 1–7. Borderline patients maintain an often fragile belief, sustained by desperate hope, that they can encounter an ideal provider in the world, yet their real-life experience has often been harsh; even in relatively good relationships, the inevitable imperfections in the other person are eventually experienced by the borderline individual as a betrayal. These patients thus come to experience all relationships with an a priori suspiciousness or paranoia. The fear of betrayal can be such that the possibility of a positive relationship is defended against (see figure 1-7) by a conscious-level insistence on the inevitability of negative interactions with others. As a result, the borderline individual is more suspicious of someone who is nice to him than he is of someone who is mean: he does not dare to believe that the niceness is real, and he apprehends meanness as a sign of being honest and "up front." The therapist's intervention may involve pointing out that the patient who insists on experiencing the therapist as negative may be defending against allowing himself a longed-for positive loving experience.

Evaluation and Treatment Contract.   In TFP the evaluation of the patient and establishment of the treatment contract are considered preparatory to ther-

FIGURE 1-7   Object-Relation Defending Against Other Dyads

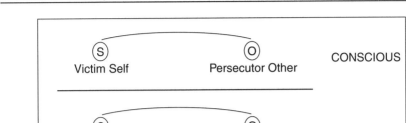

apy. It may be that the two parties cannot come to an agreement about the patient's problems and the necessary conditions of treatment. In such cases, it is appropriate to refer the patient to another form of therapy.

A thorough history must be taken to ensure that the patient is diagnosed accurately and that all information requisite to establishing an adequate treatment contract with the patient has been obtained. The contract is an essential part of the therapeutic process (Yeomans, Selzer, and Clarkin 1992). Among the conditions of treatment that the therapist must discuss with the patient are the patient's responsibilities in therapy, the therapist's responsibilities, and the particular behaviors in the patient's history that could pose a threat to the therapy.

Strategies and Tactics.   TFP strategies flow from the object relations model of borderline pathology and mandate that the therapist:

- Monitor the three channels of communication to define the dominant object relations dyads activated in the patient's relationship with the therapist
- Observe and interpret oscillations within a given dyad
- Observe and interpret connections between object relations dyads as they defend against each other, alternately keeping each other out of conscious awareness
- Encourage the integration of split-off part-objects by simultaneously increasing awareness of the split-off parts and helping the patient to see why she is keeping them split off

TFP tactics are the elements that the therapist must keep in mind to guide her through the confusion that inevitably arises on exposure to the chaos of the patient's internal world. The tactics (discussed in full in Clarkin, Yeomans, and Kernberg 1999) help keep the therapist oriented and help bring the patient's internal dynamics into focus. They entail:

- Choosing the priority theme to work with from all the material available
- Protecting the frame of treatment established in the contract, which includes the establishment of limits and the elimination of secondary gain
- Maintaining technical neutrality at most times, while also deciding when deviation from it is essential to protect the treatment
- Establishing the common ground of shared reality between therapist and patient before discussing and interpreting the patient's distortions of reality
- Analyzing both the positive and negative elements of the transference in order to avoid settling into a chronic positive (or negative) transference and splitting off the other
- Observing and analyzing primitive defenses as they appear in the transference
- Monitoring countertransference

Techniques of Transference-Focused Psychotherapy.   The techniques are the specific interventions that the therapist carries out in her interactions with the patient. The three principal interventions of TFP are:

- *Clarification:* The therapist seeks clarification from the patient about information provided by the latter that is unclear or confusing. The first phase of therapy calls for a great deal of clarification because of the confusing nature of the internal world of the borderline patient.
- *Confrontation:* Not to be confused with belligerence, confrontation consists of bringing to the patient's attention elements of his thoughts, feelings, and behaviors that seem to be contradictory. Confronting the patient with these contradictions invites him to reflect and to begin, it is hoped, to gain insight into the disparate elements of his unintegrated internal world.

- *Interpretation:* Both clarification and confrontation help prepare for effective interpretation. Interpretations make use of the information elicited through the other two techniques to link material the patient is already conscious of with inferred unconscious material believed to influence his feelings, motivation, and functioning.

Interpretations often involve helping the patient become aware of the oscillation of object relations dyads. For example, a therapist about to go on vacation might say to her patient:

You are saying that you're a victim of my mistreatment because I'm going away for two weeks, but in your actions you're yelling and screaming at me . . . basically mistreating me. I think it is difficult for you to be aware of that side of you that can be aggressive in this way because it is so distasteful for you to see any characteristics in yourself of the father you hated so much.

Interpretations also often involve pointing out that the apparently dominant object relations dyad may be defending against another object relations dyad whose impact on the patient's affective state comes from outside his awareness:

You are telling me now in a cold, detached tone that all you want to do is get strong enough to be totally independent of the rest of the world and live like a hermit who has no contact with anyone else. However, we know from previous sessions, when you were so upset that I would be leaving for two weeks, that there is a side of you that desperately wants to be close to someone and feel their warmth and support. Because of your conviction that you can never find that kind of relationship in the world, you retreat into what you are telling me now, which covers up the rest.

TFP VERSUS CONVENTIONAL
PSYCHODYNAMIC PSYCHOTHERAPY

Some experts in the field of psychotherapy argue that transference-focused psychotherapy is simply good psychodynamic psychotherapy and does not present sufficient differences from good "therapy as usual" to be considered a distinct and specific treatment model. We disagree with this view and believe the issue is not just an academic one but an important clinical one: we have found in supervising therapists on TFP that those who do not grasp the differences between TFP and conventional psychodynamic therapy have more difficulty. Clinical observation reveals correlation between a high patient dropout rate and a poorer outcome in those cases in which the therapist did not adhere to the distinctive features of TFP (that is, its modifications of standard psychodynamic therapy).

The following is an abstract of the differences between TFP and conventional psychotherapy:

- *TFP is based on a more specific treatment contract:* TFP not only puts more emphasis on the contracting process as a prerequisite to therapy but harks back to the contract more often as therapy proceeds.
- *TFP allows for deviations from technical neutrality:* These deviations may be necessitated by the patient's deviations from or attacks on the frame of the treatment–followed, once the frame is reestablished, by the therapist's return to neutrality for work with the patient to explore the meaning of the actions that necessitated the deviation.
- *TFP involves a more active role for the therapist:* This more active role may include, but is not limited to, the deviations from technical neutrality. The therapist's tone is often more intense than that of her classical psychodynamic counterpart–which is not to say that the TFP therapist is less thoughtful or reflective, but rather to emphasize that TFP interventions are geared to address in tone as well as in content the uncommonly intense affect of the borderline patient. Indeed, preliminary research findings show that skilled TFP therapists communicate quite vigorously with their patients. One consequence is that TFP therapists tend to talk more in sessions than the average psychodynamic therapist.
- *The therapist in TFP is more dependent on the nonverbal and countertransference channels of communication:* These channels are distinguished from the patient's direct verbal communications (see Clarkin, Yeomans, and Kernberg 1999). The TFP therapist must pay careful attention to the demeanor, eye gaze, tone of voice, and behaviors of the patient within the session, using them to help make inferences about activated object relations dyads that may not appear in the patient's verbal productions. The TFP therapist also

monitors her own feeling states and fantasies relating to the patient during and between sessions as a way of accessing her counter-transference. Borderline patients characteristically induce feeling states in the therapist that derive from their own part-self and part-object representations.

THE TREATMENT CONTRACT

The treatment contract in most psychodynamic therapy consists of a brief discussion of the practical parameters (scheduling sessions and paying for them), with some discussion of the method (for example, free association). By contrast, the TFP contract with borderline patients must also address all the patient behaviors identified in the evaluation sessions as potential threats to treatment. Among the most typical such behaviors are suicidal actions, self-mutilation, eating disorders, substance abuse, lying or withholding of information, and a passive, inactive lifestyle. Specific parameters must be defined to address them before the therapy begins and to contain the threat of their emergence, which could interfere with the exploration of the patient's internal world. How to establish parameters around these behaviors is discussed in detail elsewhere (Selzer, Koenigsberg, and Kernberg 1987; Yeomans, Selzer, and Clarkin 1992; Clarkin, Yeomans, and Kernberg 1999). The point is that a clearly established and mutually acceptable contract is a precondition for treatment.

The TFP therapist must be constantly attentive to breaches of the contract. Tempting as it may be to pursue some other theme at the time the breach is noted, the therapist must adhere to the TFP treatment priorities and immediately invoke the contract (Clarkin, Yeomans, and Kernberg 1999, p. 49).

The therapist might say:

> I would be very interested in the new fantasies you're experiencing when having sex with your husband, but first we have to look at what you said about having to have a drink before feeling comfortable going to bed with him. Part of your initial contract was to stay away from alcohol altogether and to attend AA meetings at least three times a week. If you're not adhering to those conditions of treatment, we have to address that. Your drinking could totally undermine our ability to work effectively in therapy, as it did in your last therapy. It also must mean something that, at this particular point in our work, you have begun to drink again. We will need to understand this.

Further, the therapist must recognize the need to add new conditions to the contract if new potentially undermining behaviors arise. For instance, when the patient has not paid the bill for two months, the therapist may not only see a threat to the continuation of the treatment but experience an impact on his countertransference. He might say:

> When we began working together, you said that you did not think you would have any problem paying for therapy. However, two months have gone by now with no payment. If there has been some change in your circumstances, I would be happy to discuss an adjustment of the fee or other options. However, if there hasn't been any change, we need to agree upon when the fee should be paid each month. After we agree on this, we can proceed to look at what this all means.

DEVIATIONS FROM TECHNICAL NEUTRALITY

Neutrality is the position from which the therapist observes the forces of the patient's id, superego, and acting ego, as well as those of external reality. Neutrality is also the position from which the therapist assists the patient's observing ego to understand the interactions of these other agencies; that treatment goal is predicated on the idea that conscious understanding helps to resolve conflicts between the forces and to reduce the symptoms associated with them (such as anxiety and depression). Accordingly, the therapist does not side with any of the agencies involved.

The TFP therapist generally remains neutral. The nature of borderline pathology is such, however, that manifestations of the patient's aggression (overt or veiled) would sometimes seriously threaten the continuation of the therapy if left unchecked. At such times, the TFP therapist may temporarily abandon neutrality; he should return to it, however, as soon as it is possible to do so and then analyze with the patient what necessitated the deviation.

In the case of a patient who announces her intention to quit her job abruptly, a therapist might normally explore the libidinal or aggressive drives involved, superego admonitions, and external elements of the job, and then work with the patient to sort out the various factors without taking a side. If both the therapist and the patient know, however, that the patient's husband pays for her therapy on the condition that she hold a job, her decision to quit would merit a different response from the therapist:

What you do in your life is up to you, but this decision has serious ramifications for therapy. You husband will pay for it only if you are working, so by talking about quitting your job, you're talking about quitting therapy. I can't tell how conscious or unconscious it is on your part—we can look at that later—but I feel it's my responsibility to advise you clearly not to do anything that would threaten our work here, which, in this case, means not quitting your job; in my opinion, the problems that brought you to therapy are still very present, and it would be a tragedy to give up the opportunity to work on them. If talking about quitting your job is an indirect way to say that you want to leave therapy, that's the issue we should be addressing.

INCREASING THE THERAPIST'S LEVEL OF ACTIVITY AND UTILIZING THE NONVERBAL AND COUNTERTRANSFERENCE CHANNELS

The TFP therapist may be very active in sessions and even, at times, between sessions. The need for this level of activity has to do with the psychic structure of the borderline individual, whose internal world is characterized by dramatically different and mutually split-off representations of self and others. Consequently, the patient may respond to the therapist in dramatically different ways at different times, depending on which internal object representation is active in his mind; since there is no integration of the split-off representations, each one exists in an extreme form and may overwhelm the patient's perception of the immediate situation.

There are times when a patient's transference is so thoroughly fixed on experiencing the therapist as a bad, dangerous, persecutory object that a logical response for the patient, *within that transference,* would be to withdraw from the therapist and the therapy, thus taking the serious risk of ending the treatment. The challenge for the therapist is to welcome this intensely negative transference but to work with it in a way that keeps the patient from reacting to it by dropping out of treatment. The therapist may therefore be very active in intervening, consistent with the mandate to work with the healthy part of the patient—no matter how small and hard to locate that part may sometimes be.

Patients organized at the borderline level often have little awareness of the inner representations that guide their interactions; they defend against deepening their conscious understanding, since doing so would threaten the internal splitting, with the resultant increased anxiety and the shattering of precious idealizations. Consequently, their verbalizations in the early phase of therapy often tend toward trivialization. The therapist must "read" the interaction in order to begin to formulate an understanding of the patient's inner world and may need to base interpretations on what the patient is doing and on his own countertransference in order to advance the treatment or avoid dropout. Operating with a relative paucity of verbal input from the patient requires the TFP therapist to intervene before the usual amount of data surfaces, and accordingly to call on object relations theory to guide him in making interpretations more often than the traditional psychotherapist does.

The therapist's increased level of activity may be reflected between sessions as well as in sessions. For example, in a classical psychodynamic psychotherapy, if a patient does not come to a session, the therapist typically waits until the next session to discuss it. In TFP, the therapist would be more likely to call the patient to inquire about what was going on because it is possible that the patient's negative representation of the therapist may have gotten the upper hand and may have led her to decide to cut off all contact with the therapist. The therapist uses his assessment of the current state of the transference to decide on the appropriate level of activity.

CHAPTER 2

Factors That Shape Borderline Personality Disorder

The model of borderline personality organization presented in the preceding chapter emphasizes the patient's maintenance of separate part-self and -object dyads that correspond to differently valenced emotional interactions with early caregivers. In the face of particularly intense affects, primitive defenses such as splitting keep these partial dyads from coalescing into more realistic wholes in order to protect idealized images from destruction. This model is useful in conceptualizing the mental schemata available to the borderline patient to apprehend and guide his interactions with others and with self. As such, it also provides a framework for understanding his interpersonal behavior and the vicissitudes of the transference, and for guiding the interpretive work of TFP.

What is less clear is *why* some individuals develop a borderline structure—that is, why they defend against the coalescing of the part dyads into integrated, realistic, whole representations. This defense is probably codetermined by multiple interacting factors and also may be a final common pathway reached by a number of different routes. For example, intense levels of aggression resulting either from inborn impairments in anger modulation or from early exposure to pain or abuse may foster the use of splitting to protect idealized objects from intense aggression.

21

Recent studies of normal and abnormal personalities have begun to shed light on some of the biological and developmental factors involved. Recognizing the complex interplay of these factors should help therapists better appreciate the mix of forces that their patients must contend with, although thus far the field has translated little of the new understanding of personality development into specific clinical strategies. To a limited degree, we have begun to apply attachment research and neurobiological findings when we address the patient's ability to connect with the therapist and when we make pharmacological interventions. These issues are discussed more fully in chapters 6 and 12.

In modern usage, the term "personality" embraces both temperament and character. Temperament refers to inborn and constitutional differences in the automatic responses of individuals to emotional or affect-laden stimuli; these responses are fortified under the influence of associative conditioning. Temperament traits are generally observable in infants and remain stable throughout life. Character and its corresponding traits are reflections of differences in early learning and in the self-teaching about life that stems from intuition, as shaped and modified by the learning individuals have absorbed from parents and important others. Cloninger, Svrakic, and Przybeck (1993) speak of character as what we make of ourselves intentionally, as distinct from temperament, which is how we are born. Of course, in reality the two interact.

The environmental factors that underlie character development also play the predominant role in the phenomenon of attachment. As we shall see in greater detail in chapter 6, the forces that determine whether a person shows secure attachment or one of the various forms of insecure attachment also affect personality development, in the same measure. We will look at the correlations that are emerging between the varieties of insecure attachment and certain disorders of personality, as they are commonly diagnosed at the clinical level.

PSYCHOBIOLOGICAL
UNDERPINNINGS OF PERSONALITY

The neurophysiologist Gerald Edelman has marshaled evidence to the effect that the brain, with its 12 billion neurons (and their quadrillion interconnections), is capable of self-organization, engaging in the same sort of evolutionary processes at the micro level that animal and plant species show at the macro level. Although the whole process continues throughout life, it is most active in infancy and early childhood.

The fine structure of the cerebral cortex is constantly in flux. Immediately after birth, experience has a profound impact on the paths taken by various neurons, the number of initially undifferentiated stem cells that transform into neurons, the number of dendritic connections, and the specific connections that are made. Optimal nurturing helps maintain the ideal volume and cell number in various key brain centers that subserve memory systems, such as the hippocampus and amygdala. The functioning of cortical centers involved with the conscious and unconscious processing of information is likewise experience-dependent: optimal nurturing and life experience promote optimal connectivity and mental processing, creating an optimal "wiring pattern."

By contrast, traumatic experiences, especially if severe, sustained, and repetitive, lead to cell damage and premature death in key centers and to wiring patterns that evoke unmodulated and maladaptive responses to the ordinary events of life. Despite the plasticity of the brain—greater in childhood than in one's older years—severe trauma of the sort that initiates a post-traumatic stress disorder (PTSD) reconfigures the brain often in an irreversible, or near-irreversible manner, diminishing the cell volume in key memory centers. The elegant work of Bessel van der Kolk (1989) has helped trace the actual pathways and brain centers activated as traumatized persons try to recollect their painful experiences. Depending on the nature and timing of their traumatic experiences, and on "host" factors having to do with the inherited architecture of their brains, such persons may develop dissociative disorders, including multiple personality or the kind of splitting that we have discussed as a signature defense mechanism in borderline personality.

Women who have been subjected to incest by a father or other older relative are especially at risk to develop both BPD as defined by *DSM-IV* and some of the symptoms associated with PTSD. For this reason, Jerome Kroll (1993) in Minnesota has asserted that BPD is just a brand of PTSD. This exaggerates the picture, since BPD is best seen as a condition that demonstrates "equifinality": different causative routes may lead to the same clinical syndrome. A trauma history is very common in hospitalized women with BPD. Clinicians working in such centers can be easily misled into forgetting that other factors may play the major role in certain BPD patients.

The interplay between focal molecular neurobiological changes and behavior is a topic currently receiving much attention. Both psychosocial stresses and bouts of affective illness (depression especially) can alter the brain in such a way as to create neurological vulnerabilities that are difficult or impossible to reverse. Persons suffering from such stress or gene abnormalities are prone to periodic outbreaks of illness or to chronic disorders of personality. Severe psychosocial stresses do not alter the genes but may alter gene expression, including the timing or force with which certain gene-driven vulnerabilities manifest at the clinical level. As R. M. Post and S. R. B. Weiss of the NIMH (1997) maintain, life-threatening trauma may set in motion neurobiological changes that continue throughout life to affect mood, behavior, sleep, arousal, and memory. After stressful life events precipitate a certain number of episodes of symptom outbreak, illness can emerge later, even without any obvious stressor.

Psychiatric conditions are, as far as we know, mostly polygenic. This means they are associated with many (abnormal) genes and their corresponding vulnerabilities, creating a picture of vast complexity. Thus, for instance, in the case of Huntington's chorea, the culprit is a single gene on the fourth chromosome (which, though present in every cell in the body, expresses itself only in the striatal cells of the brain, where it causes premature cell death), but in psychiatric conditions there is a great increase in the influence of environment and a corresponding reduction in so-called genetic determinism.

Recall Harlow's experiments in the 1950s with monkeys reared by a monkey mother versus a cloth or wire monkey (Harlow and Harlow 1963). Even a cloth surrogate mother was not enough to promote normal monkey development, a finding that paralleled Rene Spitz's (1946) observations of severely deprived infants in orphanages. We know from recent experiments in neonatal rodents (McEwen 1994) that stress, if sufficient, leads to increased death of hippocampal neurons, correlating with later performance deficits; the same sequence occurs with high levels of cortisol, like those found in the bloodstream of depressed persons (cf. McEwen, Gould, and Sakai 1992). In other animal experiments, repeated periods of maternal deprivation led to prolonged increase in blood cortisol (again as in human depression). The maternally deprived animals were unusually prone to ingest cocaine or alcohol (Plotsky and Meany 1993), as is the case with borderline, antisocial, and other severely personality-disordered persons, among whom maternal deprivation and other early traumata are commonplace (as is self-medication with such drugs).

The effects of optimal nurturing—good mothering—are the reverse. Enriched early environments are associated with an increased number of synapses and dendritic connections. Moreover, in the optimally nurtured young more stem cells differentiate into neurons (Gage et al. 1995). This means, in effect, that optimal environmental complexity becomes mirrored in heightened CNS complexity. Furthermore, L. X. Zhang and his colleagues (1997) have shown that even brief maternal deprivation (in animals) leads to increased cell death in the hippocampus, meaning that deprivation could lead to permanent changes for the worse in the developing nervous system. Acute stressors (like physical abuse or incest), in contrast to neglect, may leave indelible memory traces, as noted earlier in the case of PTSD; these involve (adverse) emotional memories, processed by the amygdala. Children exposed to both neglect and abuse are presumably prone to both underdevelopment of hippocampus- and amygdala-mediated memory systems and permanent "branding" of painful memories in the cortex. In addition, they are likely to have a "kindled" nervous system, that is, one prone to overreact even to mild stimuli that happen to be reminiscent of the original traumata.

The research of Larry Siever and his colleagues (1999) has contributed importantly to our understanding of the psychobiological underpinnings of borderline disorder. J. M. Silverman and his colleagues (1991), for example, found that the *relatives* of borderline patients, when compared with the relatives of schizophrenics or patients with other personality disorders, showed a greater number of affective and impulsive personality traits, although not a greater likelihood of major affective disorder. Their results suggested that there is familial transmission of two of the key traits of BPD patients—namely, affective instability and impulsivity—and that these traits may be to an extent genetically independent.

In another study, A. S. New and her colleagues (1999) noted decreased serum cholesterol levels–a finding already observed in certain persons with impulsive aggression–in borderline patients when compared to nonborderline patients. In still another study, B. J. Steinberg and his colleagues (1997) found that there is a greater depressive response to physostigmine challenge (operating on the cholinergic system) in borderline patients than in nonborderline patients, suggesting that the cholinergic system may play a role in affect regulation.

In addition, Siever and his colleagues (1999), in their study of the serotonergic system in personality-disordered patients, have shown that borderline individuals have a tendency toward reduced prolactin response to fenfluramine challenge. Siever and coworkers (1999a) have found that in inhibitory regions of the cortex (more specifically, the orbito-frontal area) there is less response to agents that increase serotonergic activity in impulsive (particularly borderline) patients; genes related to the serotonergic system, such as the 5HT 1b gene, also appear to be related to impulsive aggression. These findings, in turn, offer a rationale for the use of serotonin-reuptake blockers such as fluoxetine (Prozac), as well as mood-stabilizing medications, in the treatment of borderline patients. The application of the emerging biologic findings about BPD to its pharmacotherapy is discussed more fully in chapter 12.

ATTACHMENT: NEUROPHYSIOLOGY AND IMPACT ON PERSONALITY

Over the last ten years, research in animal and human neurophysiology and in attachment theory has developed to the point where some integration across fields is becoming possible. This in turn is contributing to a better understanding of personality development. The infant, for example, coevolves with its "environment"—at first primarily its mother, or "caregiver" (or, in Kohut's [1971] terminology, "self-object"). The environmental factors that underlie character development play the predominant role in the phenomenon of attachment: the brain's self-organizing systems are capable of generating new internal representations in response to changing environmental conditions.

The fluctuations in the early mother-infant environment are amplified by emotion, which serves as a catalyst to self-organization (Schore 1994). Attachment patterns arise through the consolidation of the interpretations the infant makes about mother and her changing responses. These interpretations—at first necessarily nonverbal, more like "impressions"—are woven into the infant's "working model" of its environment. Mothers and babies look at each other a great deal, and their synchronized gazes lead to changes in the infant's bodily (and brain) states; the mother, in effect, regulates the infant's autonomic nervous system. This brings about a mutual entrainment of both their central nervous systems. Attachment experiences represent affective transactions in which the mother modulates her infant's arousal level.

In face-to-face interactions, the mother's gaze has the effect of stimulating corticotropin releasing factor (CRF) in the infant's paraventricular hypothalamus. Plasma noradrenalin increases. The sympathetic nervous system is activated. The end result is emotional excitement. Other effects include the release of endorphins and ACTH and the activation of the ventral tegmental system, leading to dopamine release and the emotion of elation. Dopamine receptors in the prefrontal cortex, thus activated, promote memory, learning, and cognitive processes. These events in the infant's brain are thus experience-dependent—as are the increasing size and complexity of the dendritic arbors and of synaptic connections—when mother and infant are well attuned and comfortable with one another. In the ideal state, this rapid neural activity in the infant is associated with imprinting, rapid learning, and optimal formation of attachment bonds: "Cells that fire together wire together" (Post and Weiss 1997).

During the first five years of life, but especially in the first two, the brain undergoes the selective loss of synapses and dendritic connections in pathways that are no longer of much usefulness. (This is why the neuronal wiring adapts so exclusively to the "mother tongue" that after age twelve one can no longer learn to speak a foreign language without an accent.) The self-organizing brain becomes increasingly in tune with its environment. The mother's behavior serves as the agent of "natural selection" at the micro level, shaping her infant's developing self. Self-organization is therefore initially a two-person process.

In early infancy, before most of the cortex is myelinated, the amygdala are dominant in shaping the infant's emotional life. By the end of the first year, the orbito-insular region of the prefrontal cortex—which responds to faces—plays an important role in interpreting signals related to social interaction. Specifically, the orbito-frontal cortex processes the rapid visual and auditory scanning of the mother's emotionally expressive face and speech. Information thus gathered unconsciously guides the infant's behavior. As a control center for emotion, the orbito-frontal cortex acts as an analog amplifier. Tiny inputs (the mother's slight smile or frown, for example) can trigger major changes in output, causing dramatic shifts in affect. In unfavorable mother-infant situations, the infant loses the ability to overcome negative affects quickly. Negative affects induced in the infant (by a mother who is chronically critical or hostile, for example) take a long time to diminish to baseline level. This pattern of remaining in a state of emergency or fear for much longer than usual is characteristic of persons with borderline personality.

The orbital prefrontal cortex is more voluminous on the right side, which may account for its primacy in the reading of emotion (be it high arousal, like terror, excitement, or elation, or low arousal, like shame). The right cerebral cortex processes faces, and since the left face is read by the right cortex of the viewer, it is not surprising that the left side of a face shows more emotion than the right side. The right hemisphere is thus centrally involved in human bonding and attachment; the left is more concerned with the less powerful emotions, like interest, guilt, or enjoyment. Gene-environment mechanisms are embedded in face-to-face emotional interactions: the mother acts as the hidden regulator of the infant's emotion-processing circuitry (amygdala, limbic system, orbito-frontal cortex).

Maternal deprivation can cause long-lasting abnormalities in social-emotional function. It may be associated with a decrease in dopaminergic neurons in the ventral tegmental area. Disturbed mother-infant relations create in this way a biological substrate for heightened vulnerability to despair and depression, whereas optimal mothering with good attunement brings about a modulation of the infant's cortisol-mediated response to stress. The normal infant shows a quicker return of cortisol to baseline levels—that is, a more resilient coping mechanism. Excessively high cortisol levels, in contrast, inhibit dendritic branching, prompt synaptic destruction in emotional centers in the limbic system, and thus lead to permanent impairment in the adaptive handling of emotions.

Michael Rutter and his colleagues (1997) make the point that environmental stresses—such as poor attunement between mother and child, or abusive parent-child patterns—exert their most severe impact on children who come "prepared" for trouble because of genetic susceptibility to one or another psychological disorder. Such children are especially at risk to develop dysfunction in the right orbito-frontal cortex. This is noted in a wide variety of conditions, including schizophrenia, uni- and bipolar illness, addiction to drugs or alcohol, and also in borderline, narcissistic, and psychopathic personalities.

Another problem that can arise is impairment in social perception, meaning difficulty in evaluating facial expressions, gestures, and speech prosody. Such impairment, which may be a response to severe stress in early childhood, leads to extreme right frontal hyperactivity, with excessive emotional reactions to even mild stresses later on, and this can lead to introversion of personality, schizoid traits, or to a decreased ability to display affect (as in severe cases of obsessive-compulsive personality).

In general, an infant born with genetic coding for abnormal neurophysiological reactions who is paired with a mother who is poorly attuned will develop a cortico-limbic organization that copes poorly with stressful situations. As Schore points out, such a neural organization becomes static, closed, and heavily invested in defensive structures to guard against interpersonal experiences that the individual anticipates would trigger painful emotions and mental disorganization.

With regard to gene-environment interplay in general, contemporary research (Bouchard 1994) suggests that about half the variance in personality features can be considered genetic. The majority of people have little genetic risk for a major psychiatric illness. Those fortunate enough to have well-attuned mothers and abuse-free upbringings will show only minor peculiarities of personality, reflecting mostly genetic or constitutional, rather than environmental, differences. Gender, which is genetically determined and shaped further by intrauterine conditions, can be one such difference: men are more likely to show obsessive traits (including isolation of affect, for example), and women the so-called hysteric traits (such as, at a subclinical level, greater emotional responsivity).

Some persons, of course, are born with a high genetic-constitutional predisposition to emotional disorder, including personality disorder.[1] Even a consistently nurturing mother cannot protect totally against an eventual outbreak in such cases. But good nurturing may attenuate its severity, and the result may be a mildly schizoid, mildly paranoid, mildly depressive personality. Alternatively, infants with extreme genetic loading for, say, schizoid or autistic conditions may, because of their inborn handicaps in

---

[1]To demonstrate better the interplay of genetic and environmental factors, Irving Gottesman and his colleagues (Goldsmith, Gottesman, and Lemery 1997) have offered a reaction-surface model. Using a cube diagram, environment is placed along one axis (ranging from "protective" to "hazardous"). Genotype is placed along another, ranging from "resistant" to "susceptible." The risk for antisocial behavior, for example, is zero in the presence of resistant genotype and protective environment. But the risk is almost inescapable where susceptible genotype meets the most hazardous environment.

forming attachments, actually alienate mothers with the potential for attunement and nurturing. A vicious circle may develop whereby the mother becomes tense and intolerant, feels guilt-ridden (a "failure"), and inadvertently intensifies the child's preexisting disability in attachment development. A rare phenomenon is the child whose genetic predisposition to extremely low empathy (perhaps on the basis of low cell volume in the right orbito-frontal cortex) is combined with low serotonin in key pathways related to impulsive aggression; such a child may become a psychopath, even if raised by what D. W. Winnicott (1965) would have called a good-enough mother. (This scenario probably explains the few cases in the forensic literature of psychopathic criminals from approximately normal backgrounds.)

ATTACHMENT STYLES AND PERSONALITY DISORDERS, ESPECIALLY BORDERLINE

Contemporary interest in attachment styles, and the related research, were stimulated by the pioneering work of John Bowlby (1969) and by the diagnostic and classification system developed by Mary Main (1995). The four styles elaborated by Main, which are discussed more fully in chapter 6, are the free/autonomous (or secure), the dismissive (or avoidant), the preoccupied (or ambivalent), and the unresolved (or fearful).[2] Dismissive persons tend to derogate others and to cut themselves off from close attachment. The preoccupied are typically passively angry and entangled with intimates (such as mother originally, and sexual partners now). The unresolved, in adult life, show signs of disorganization when the original attachment figure is discussed; Peter Fonagy and his colleagues (1996) speculate that the unresolved person may have been abused by the attachment figure yet feels overwhelming guilt and fear when talking about the experience.

---

[2]It now appears that different types of attachment abnormalities are associated with different types of connectional degeneration. Chronically abused infants with disorganized, insecure attachment show particularly high cortisol levels and also respond to threats with long-lasting elevation of sympathetic amines. Insecure attachment of the resistant (dismissive) type is associated with expansion of the excitatory ventral tegmental circuit. The resultant psychopathology tends to be of the "externalizing" type. Insecure avoidant attachment is associated with an expanded lateral tegmental circuitry—which is inhibitory. The tendency is toward internalization of painful affects.

Daniel Stern (1999), who found in his study of infants that the attachment style at twelve months is the best predictor of behavior at age five or six (1999), suggested that the fearful or avoidant child tends to act, when separated briefly from mother, as though she "didn't matter." This reduction of affective signaling optimizes the distance between infant and mother, since the mother would be rejecting if the infant were to attempt too much closeness (too much for her comfort). The preoccupied infant tends to amplify the signal (through crying, for example) in order to maximize the chance that the mother will notice it and begin to soothe it. This latter style is common in those who go on to develop borderline personality disorder.

Fonagy speaks also of the reflective function (RF), the capacity to reflect on one's own mental state, which can be assessed via a questionnaire and a corresponding scale. As Fonagy and Higgitt (1989) showed in their study of personality-disordered patients, those with BPD (using the *DSM-IV* definition) usually exhibited the preoccupied style. This was true, though to a lesser extent, of patients with paranoid and other disorders (some of whom showed the dismissive style). Six out of ten patients with an abuse history were diagnosed with BPD; only one in seven without such a history was diagnosed with BPD. But almost all of those who had an abuse history coupled with low RF ability were diagnosed with BPD, whereas only one in six of the abused persons with high RF was also borderline. In psychoanalytic terms, Fonagy characterizes the BPD patient as someone who is likely to have been a victim of abuse or neglect, who usually has low reflective function, and who shows a preoccupied attachment style, often with poor resolution of the early abuse experiences.

Fonagy and his colleagues (1995) have also studied the interplay between parents and their young children. Focusing on the influence of parental mental representations on the infant's behavior in stressful situations, they concluded that parents who rated high in reflective function were about four times as likely to have children with secure attachment as were parents who rated low. A few of the children whose parents had the highest ratings were nevertheless insecure in their attachment, indicating that they were innately more vulnerable to psychopathology.

Fonagy favors a new dialectic model of object relations in which the infant internalizes the caregiver's evolving image of him and the internalization becomes the core of the child's "mentalizing self." (Fonagy's interpersonal model parallels the neurobiological paradigm that spotlights the interaction of the limbic system and the orbito-frontal cortex in both mother and infant.) He speaks also of how an abusive or hostile relationship with the mother may lead the infant to turn away from its "mentalizing object" (mother) because the infant registers the mother's hatred or indifference. The infant will tend to react with a disavowal of mental states, with the unfortunate result that his chances of establishing intimate links with a more understanding person later on are reduced (Fonagy et al. 1995, p. 258). The child becomes therefore at risk of developing one of several personality disorders—paranoid, narcissistic, or obsessive-compulsive. Under extreme conditions, the child's fear of his mother's mind can have "devastating consequences on the emergence of social understanding" (p. 258) and may contribute to the development of borderline personality—which is usually charcterized by disordered, short-lived, chaotic, and intense attachments (p. 259).

The importance of the reflective function shows itself in the Adult Attachment Interviews (AAIs) of BPD patients, who exhibited a common pattern: high prevalence of sexual abuse, low RF, and lack of resolution of the abuse. It suggested that children who were maltreated and who responded to their maltreatment with an inhibition of reflective function were less likely to resolve the abuse and, as a consequence, more likely to reenact the abusive patterns and become "borderline." This is in line with both van der Kolk's model of trauma reenactment in BPD and the neurobiological theories mentioned earlier: trauma can harm the limbic system of the child (through synaptic destruction, cell death in the hippocampus, and so on), rendering the child less able to cope effectively with the abusive experiences.

Borderline persons with abuse histories are also likely to have developed masochistic reaction patterns. The child processes the caregiver's unfair attacks as somehow "justified" and internalizes the blame, becoming, as Fonagy and his colleagues (1995) observe, "deeply attached to the persecutor as the only path to a sense of security" (p. 268). This is, of course, a false security, because it requires molding oneself to the whims and accusations of the persecutor, whom the child now mistakes for a "normal" person who had every right to treat the child with cruelty. This situation is reminiscent of the one depicted years ago by Harry Stack Sullivan (1962/1974), who spoke of the terrible compromise of the schizophrenic when, as a child, he had to switch from thinking "bad mother" to "bad me."

PERSONALITY ORGANIZATION

Although there is no one-to-one mapping between each personality disorder and this or that attachment style, we can safely say that persons with any (severe) personality disorder show an insecure attachment pattern of some type. A final common pathway of the multiplicity of factors that can shape borderline personality is a particular structuring of the internal representations of self and others that we described in chapter 1. This fragmented structure is maintained by means of primitive defenses. Such a psychostructural description forms the basis for the personality organization classification proposed by Otto Kernberg (1967).

Locating personality disorders within the overarching framework of personality organization is helpful as a first-order guide to a treatment approach. Knowing the personality organization tells us the principal defense mechanisms and the level of reality testing available to the patient. These factors are crucial in determining whether the patient is amenable to a psychodynamic approach, and if so, which approach. If reality testing is grossly impaired, as it is in the psychotic organization, then we would not expect the patient to benefit by merely gaining conscious awareness of his internal representations; being unable to check them against reality, he would still be unable to correct them. Such a patient would be unlikely to tolerate the extended periods in psychodynamic therapy of exploration without reality feedback. If reality testing is intact, as in the borderline and neurotic organizations, psychodynamic work is, in principle, possible. When primitive defenses predominate, as in the borderline organization, then an approach that surfaces and integrates split object relations dyads and protects the treatment frame against acting out, as in TFP, may be particularly valuable. In neurotic organization, where the defense mechanisms are more mature, a psychodynamic approach with less structure, including psychoanalysis, is possible. Psychotic-level patients need supportive therapy and (usually) medications.

Patients with BPD fit into the middle (borderline organization) level, as do almost all schizotypal patients. Some personality configurations straddle more than one layer. Thus, there are hysteric persons who function at the neurotic level, but also hysteric persons who function at the borderline level. The latter have the characteristics of the *DSM-IV*'s "histrionic P.D." There are also some hysteric persons with what used to be called hysterical psychosis, meaning an individual, perhaps schizoaffective or schizophrenic, whose personality coloration is hysteric.

Even among patients with a borderline organization, some present particular challenges to TFP. This book examines some of the personality factors that impede standard TFP and considers when to emphasize particular aspects of the personality, when to pay attention to attachment style, when to integrate medication into the treatment, and when to use nonpsychodynamic approaches in preparation or as an alternative to TFP. We turn first to a review of an all too common situation: TFP is misapplied because the patient has been misdiagnosed as borderline.

CHAPTER 3

Treatment Dilemmas Arising from Misdiagnoses

In developing an approach for the "difficult" borderline patient, one of the first factors to consider is the correctness and completeness of the diagnosis. Clinicians pass along to their colleagues in training a simple yet often overlooked truth: when patients worsen or fail to respond to one or a few trials of accepted treatments, the original diagnosis should be reassessed. This issue is particularly germane for those who treat borderline patients, because nonborderline patients are often misdiagnosed as borderline. Some patients treated with TFP do not respond because they are not borderline patients, and others have unrecognized comorbid conditions that render them unsuitable for TFP. Unfortunately, neither misdiagnoses of nonborderline patients as borderline nor neglect of overriding comorbidities is uncommon in clinical practice.

Like a number of important medical disorders, borderline personality disorder is a great pretender, presenting with a wide range of symptoms that can occur in many psychiatric disorders. These include mood, anxiety, somatoform, pan-neurotic, and even psychotic symptoms such as hallucinations or delusions. If BPD can mimic such a variety of other conditions, it is not surprising that clinicians may diagnose it erroneously.

Moreover, BPD has come to be considered synonymous with dramatic impulsivity, self-destructiveness, anger, and tumultuous interpersonal relationships in spite of the fact that any of these features can be the product of a variety of other disorders. Impulsivity and self-destructiveness in particular are so prevalent among borderline patients that many clinicians consider them "signature" characteristics whose very presence "makes" the diagnosis. Clinicians sometimes apply the borderline label (especially borderline personality *disorder*) too hastily in the face of these supposedly pathognomonic features, which in fact could have arisen only rarely, or even just once, in the life of the patient (the "one swallow does not make a summer" error). The diagnosis depends, in other words, on a pattern of repeated episodes over time.

Since borderline patients have acquired a reputation for being demanding and manipulative, some clinicians also tend to assume that any controlling or difficult-to-manage patient is borderline. This is not the case. Borderline patients by no means have a monopoly on orneriness. For example, the primitive defenses of omnipotent control and projective identification, the defense mechanisms that give the appearance of manipulativeness, are found in patients with psychotic personality organization as well as those with borderline organization. Individuals may also act manipulatively simply because they are willing to achieve a goal through devious means. They may be dishonest exploiters, but not necessarily personality-disordered. Nevertheless, such patients are often labeled borderline.

Even evidence of classic symptoms of a psychotic illness, such as hallucinations or paranoid delusions, may not dissuade some clinicians from making a borderline diagnosis instead because such symptoms are occasionally seen (albeit transiently) in borderline patients. Thus, owing to the array of symptoms that the diagnosis can absorb, it is not unusual for better-functioning schizophrenic patients, bipolar I patients, malingerers, patients with factitious disorders, or even criminals to be mislabeled borderline. Treated with TFP, such individuals may show no change, regress, or simply exploit the process.

A corresponding clinical error relates more to treatment than to diagnosis. The patient may meet the criteria for a borderline disorder by one of the accepted diagnostic methods, but if the borderline features are grossly overshadowed by the features of another personality disorder or another condition, the patient may be inaccessible to TFP. Patients with antisocial personality, for instance, are not considered candidates for TFP, although it is possible that some with antisocial features may respond to it. (See chapter 5 for a more complete discussion of the extent to which antisocial traits in a borderline patient can be treated.)

Another relative contraindication for TFP is secondary gain from the symptomatic behavior, which is prominent when BPD is comorbid with malingering or factitious illness and cannot be relinquished. In such situations, therapists may apply treatment methods that are valid for the "textbook" borderline patient, in whom the borderline organization or the BPD items are paramount, downplaying the importance of some other personality disorder or symptom complex that happens to dominate, often glaringly, the overall clinical picture.

Mistakes of these kinds are common in forensic psychiatry. Therapists in institutions may be eager to see certain patients in a more favorable light than circumstances warrant, and a diagnosis of BPD may help them to maintain a measure of optimism that makes their difficult work easier to bear. It may also affirm that they know what to do: if the patient is "borderline," that is a condition in which they have had considerable training. Such mistakes occur in private practice settings as well, typically when some quality of the patient activates "rescue fantasies" in the countertransference, or when the patient's powerful use of projective identification independently instills a grandiose rescuer image in the therapist.

SCHIZOPHRENIA MISDIAGNOSED AS BORDERLINE PERSONALITY DISORDER

Some schizophrenic patients mutilate or otherwise injure themselves in ways that are at once flamboyant and grotesque. Such acts push their self-destructive behavior into the limelight, obscuring or deemphasizing the many other signs and symptoms of their underlying psychosis. As a result, clinicians are sometimes misled into thinking that BPD is the primary diagnosis, especially if the schizophrenic patient, despite delusory ideation, does not have a formal thought disorder and therefore talks in a "rational" fashion.

One of the more striking such instances known to the authors concerns a man in his early twenties who had begun to decompensate when he was about eighteen. Having received an influenza vaccine that had become painful, he conceived the idea of getting rid of the offending arm by walking into the bear cage at the local zoo in the hope that the bear would eat the arm, thus eliminating the pain. The unobliging animal merely scratched him up a bit, at which point the authorities rescued him and transported him to a psychiatric facility. While there, the man, unprovoked, bit off part of the ear of another patient and was transported once again, this time to a forensic center where he could be better managed. There he was noted to entertain the delusion that he was pregnant. For the most part, he was calm and cooperative on the unit and seemed rational enough—so long as the subject of pregnancy was not brought up. But periodically he would become agitated and attempt to escape, climbing up the hospital fence, which was topped with razor-wire. He cut himself a number of times in this way, necessitating many stitches. Because of this impulsive self-destructiveness, he was considered by some a borderline patient (admittedly an unusually dramatic one) and by others a schizophrenic patient with BPD. But he showed none of the other features of BPD: he was not inordinately angry (though he became aggressive during his bouts of agitation), not affectively labile, and not involved in stormy interpersonal relationships. His conviction that he was pregnant might be seen as evidence of an "identity disturbance," but it was best understood as a manifestation of his schizophrenic psychosis. (In any case, even two positive items do not clinch a diagnosis of BPD.) He did respond to high-dose neuroleptics and mood stabilizers (such that the episodes of agitation disappeared), but he remained quite unreachable through verbal psychotherapy.

BIPOLAR I DISORDER
MISDIAGNOSED AS BPD

Depending on the patient sample, a fair number of patients with BPD are "comorbid" for bipolar I or bipolar II disorder (Koenigsberg et al., 1999). This may be because BPD falls along a bipolar spectrum, as Hagop S. Akiskal (1981) has proposed; because a biological vulnerability to affective instability predisposes to both bipolar and borderline conditions; or because overlapping diagnostic criteria make it easier for patients to merit diagnoses in both categories. Nevertheless, when patients meet criteria for both Axis I bipolar disorder and BPD, it is not unusual for the Axis I diagnosis to be missed and the patient to be treated as borderline. The impulsivity, grandiosity, irritability, and anger of the bipolar patient are ascribed to the borderline pathology. When the interpersonal symptoms are sufficiently florid, such signs of bipolar disorder as decreased need for sleep, pressured speech, or manic behavior may be overlooked. The clinical difficulties here are that the patient does not receive mood-stabilizing medication and that psychotherapy is undertaken in a patient with flight of ideas, a thought disorder, and manic delusions.

One such patient was a thirty-five-year-old attorney who had been hired by a successful woman investment banker to finalize a deal. After the business transaction was completed, they had a brief sexual relationship. When the attorney was rebuffed, he could not accept the rejection and began to call the woman repeatedly; when the calls were not returned, the attorney telephoned her business partners. Finally, the investment banker called the police and the harassment stopped—but some six months later the calls spontaneously resumed, occurring at all times of the day and night. The attorney's calls became threatening, and he was arrested and placed on probation, until his bad judgment (or psychotic grandiosity) got the upper hand and he announced to his probation officer that he was going to kill the investment banker—whereupon he was promptly jailed.

In jail the attorney became agitated, made a suicide gesture, and was psychiatrically evaluated and diagnosed with borderline personality disorder. His virtual stalking of the investment banker was taken as evidence of an intolerance of aloneness; the threats as evidence of excessive anger; and the suicide attempt as a classic borderline symptom. At the urging of the prosecutor, the patient was transferred to a long-term borderline treatment unit, and it was there, where his behavior could be directly observed on a twenty-four-hour basis, that the correct diagnosis of bipolar I disorder was made. The patient's speech was pressured, he was grandiose, and he did not need to sleep, remaining up all night singing and shouting for days on end. Convinced that the psychiatrist was his enemy, he decided to stop speaking to him, against his attorney's advice that he cooperate. In other words, he displayed features of a full-blown manic episode.

WHEN CRIMINALITY IS CONFUSED WITH OR OVERSHADOWS BORDERLINE PATHOLOGY

Antisocial Personality with Psychopathic Features Masquerading as Borderline

A woman in her midtwenties was referred for transference-focused psychotherapy because of a condition thought to be borderline with depressive comorbidity. This was an accurate reading of her level of organization, though in the totality of her personality aberrations the borderline features were less worrisome and much less prominent than were the antisocial features. The daughter of a well-respected minister, she had been raised in a home free of both neglect and abuse. On both her parents' parts there was love without pampering, and the inculcation of moral values without punitiveness. She felt uncomfortable, nevertheless, growing up in a "fishbowl" where her actions were more carefully scrutinized by outsiders because of her background. She resented her parents partly on this account, and partly on the grounds that they were not as well off as the families of her fellow students at the private school she had attended.

By the time she was in her early twenties, she had become markedly vain, moody, and envious. Being unable to get a Gucci bag or Ferragamo shoes, as her friends easily could, was a hammer-blow to her ego. To rectify this "injustice," she took to stealing her parents' credit cards, running up clothing bills in the high thousands. She was persuaded to see a therapist, but only for a few weeks; thereafter, she made extended coast-to-coast calls to a guru she had heard about, running up phone bills as high as her clothing bills. In desperation, her parents locked her out of their house, though they continued to pay for her apartment. This was the point at which she was referred for TFP.

She presented herself as depressed at first, but it became apparent that she could turn tears off and on for effect and that the sadness was not genuine. What was genuine was her rage against her parents for not welcoming her back into the family and for not forgiving her debts. Her motivation for therapy was nil, except insofar as she could manipulate the therapist into arguing her "case" before her parents; when he refused to play defense attorney, he became another enemy.

Never on time for her appointments (for which her parents were paying) even at the beginning, she began skipping most of her sessions, or coming when there were only five or ten minutes left. At the family meeting that ensued, she took the opportunity to hurl curses at all and started to storm out of the office. When the therapist urged her to calm down and discuss the situation rationally, she said: "If you try to block my way, I'll kill you!" She quit treatment shortly afterward. Her behavior remained unchanged; several months later, she was arrested for credit card fraud.

Her complex personality profile contained antisocial, narcissistic, histrionic, and borderline traits (including five BPD criteria—stormy relations, anger, labile affect, boredom, and impulsivity). Her antisociality, the major area of disturbance, was accompanied by many of Robert D. Hare's Factor-I or narcissistic psychopathic traits (Hare et al. 1990): superficial charm, grandiosity, conning, manipulativeness, deceitfulness, lack of empathy or remorse, and failure to take responsibility for her actions. Like many persons (especially women) from middle- or upper-class homes, she was not a juvenile delinquent: she had not been arrested for a variety of crimes and had thus not violated parole. Her score on the Psychopathy Checklist (twenty items that can be rated 0, 1, or 2) fell short of the 30 used in the United States and Canada as diagnostic of psychopathy—exposing the limitation of the scoring system for certain populations, since she was as psychopathic as many a person scoring higher, but more shielded than most. As is typical of psychopathic persons, and in keeping with Hare's observation (1993) about people with her personality configuration, she was contemptuous of psychiatry and saw nothing wrong with her personality—qualities that combine to defeat the efforts of therapists.

BPD Misdiagnosed in a Female Sexual Offender

A woman of twenty-eight had been remanded to a forensic hospital in the wake of an episode in which she sexually molested her young niece. When the woman herself was young—nine or ten years old—an uncle had begun to force sex on her, progressing to intercourse when she was a few years older. She was placed in foster care at fourteen as a result of the incest, but by that time she had already begun to abuse alcohol and street drugs (including hallucinogens). Continued heavy substance abuse induced in her a chimerical "schizophrenia," characterized by illusions, paranoid ideas, and occasional hallucinations (in which she heard only her name being called). Throughout her teen years and beyond, she was bisexual. After the breakup of one romantic relationship, she cut her forearm—the only instance of self-cutting in her life. She maintained contact with her parents after the foster-care years and acknowledged that she often got into arguments with her mother. On a few occasions, these arguments progressed to assaultiveness of a mild type: striking her mother on the back. When evaluated initially at the hospital, she was diagnosed as having both schizophrenia and BPD.

Her subsequent course did not justify either impression. Once the psychotomimetic drugs were out of her system (she was also treated with neuroleptics), the psychotic signs that had triggered the schizophrenia diagnosis disappeared. Careful assessment of the personality dimension made it clear that she actually met only a few of the BPD criteria: her anger seemed confined to her relationships with her mother and uncle; the self-cutting was an isolated episode; and even the identity disturbance item was questionable, because she felt neither confused nor upset about her bisexuality. Since she did not meet criteria for schizophrenia or BPD, antisocial personality disorder or psychopathy, her condition was more properly thought of as an impulse disorder (which might never have surfaced had she not chronically abused drugs and alcohol).

MALINGERING AND FACTITIOUS DISORDERS MASQUERADING AS OR ASSOCIATED WITH BORDERLINE PERSONALITY

MALINGERING

Malingering involves the use of illness, real, magnified, or feigned, for the purpose of either evading some unpleasant consequence or gaining medical care and comfort to which one would not otherwise have been entitled. A common goal in malingering might be to avoid army induction—by such devices as shooting oneself in the foot or drinking enormous quantities of sugared beverages just before a urine test, so as to appear diabetic.

At New York's Bellevue Hospital, impoverished men who lived on the streets used to complain of severe "back pain" in order to be hospitalized in the winter months. Men already in the hospital, if recovering on the tuberculosis ward in January and about to be discharged, would get their buddies with active TB to spit into their sputum cups; testing "positive" bought them another two months on the unit, guaranteeing that they could stay in a warm place until springtime. One does not see this kind of gross malingering very often in the psychiatric hospital, since most patients prefer to avoid the stigma attaching to mental illness. Most also do not like the side effects of the antipsychotic medications they are asked to take for their pretend schizophrenia, the illness most likely to be feigned by the psychiatric malingerer, who believes (often correctly) that he can fool the staff by claiming to hear voices, for instance, or to have delusions of Martians tape-recording his thoughts.

This kind of malingering is most likely to be encountered in the forensic hospital (as a way of avoiding prison) or in prison itself (as a way of getting to the generally pleasanter environment of the forensic hospital). Still, there are some patients outside the forensic system who resort to malingering in order to gain admission to a psychiatric hospital. The immediate goal may be to escape an intolerable home situation.

Psychosis, especially schizophrenia, is easiest to feign since the burden is on the clinician to prove that the patient does *not* hear voices or is *not* experiencing persecutory delusions. To mimic formal thought disorder would be difficult, but this is not an obligatory item in the usual classificatory systems for schizophrenia. Pretending to have a personality disorder is more difficult still, since the manifestations are more pervasive and subtle than what is involved in pretending to be "crazy."

Then there is the whole question of how *conscious* the deception is. Diagnosticians are reluctant to invoke the notion of malingering in a patient who is not clearly conscious of the desire to hoodwink the medical establishment. Travin and Protter (1984) discuss the whole spectrum of deceitful behaviors involving illness, weighing whether the patient is intentionally fooling others (the malingerer) or primarily fooling himself and imagining he is fooling others (as in factitious illness).

It is not at all common for patients to fake borderline personality, but it does occur. One such case was a fifteen-year-old girl who was admitted to a psychiatric hospital some years ago after having cut her wrists. She came from a family of high-ranking Mafiosi and had been subjected to incestuous relations with both her father and her uncle. The uncle was shot to death, in her presence, apparently by a rival gang member. There was no way she could go to the authorities and complain about the sexual violation, lest she meet a worse fate at the hands of her father. But to be "suicidal" was an acceptable means of escaping this intolerable environment. She had plenty of reason to feel genuinely distraught over what was happening, without having to *pretend* suicidality. Yet it was the impression of the hospital staff that her wrist-cutting was neither a cunning maneuver to extricate herself from the deplorable home situation nor a totally unconsciously motivated symptom expressing her despair. It was a mixture of both.

A malingerer evaluated in a forensic hospital had been hospitalized in a conventional psychiatric facility a few months earlier. There he had been treated for "depression with suicidality and borderline personality." A homeless man in his forties, he had spoken, tearfully, of how his wife and two children had been killed by stray bullets in the midst of a gangland gun feud on April 10, along with four other victims, "plus thirteen wounded."

This tragedy took the wind out of his sails, causing him to give up his job as a cook and to take to drink—and to make attempts on his life. Or so he said. His arms bore the marks of self-cutting. Treated with antidepressants, he made a gradual recovery and was discharged. Unbeknownst to the staff who had worked him up at that hospital, he had actually been arrested for selling a small amount of cocaine shortly before. He sold a larger amount after his discharge, and the second arrest had led to his transfer to the forensic hospital, because of his "serious depression." But he looked sad only in the presence of staff members, and something didn't seem right about his story. Investigation revealed that there had been no massacre in the town he identified on April 10, or on any other date within living memory. There was no record of anyone with his name or the names of his wife and daughters (in reality, he had no wife or daughters) or any of his thirteen siblings (three of whom were "Will," "Willie," and "William," because his parents "ran out of names for boys"). He had gone to the trouble of memorizing matching names and addresses of people throughout the South, but none of them had ever heard of him. His major goal was to sidestep the unpleasantness of prison by posing as the suicidally depressed survivor of a family wiped out by violence. His ingenuity earned him a spot (briefly as it turned out) as a depressed borderline in a forensic hospital, with its humanistic staff, swimming pool, basketball courts, and meticulous dietitians. The more accurate diagnosis here would be malingering in a person with antisocial personality.

A less artful malingerer, also admitted to the forensic hospital after a drug arrest, had a longer arrest record, mostly for drug-related offenses, but had now been remanded to a forensic hospital as a "schizophrenic." The schizophrenia had been diagnosed at the time of his last arrest, when he had given voice to "delusions"—especially that of being the great-great-grandson of a famous Hollywood actor, who in reality was only a little older than the patient. He also spoke of graduating from high school with marks so high that they earned him "automatic medical and law degrees" and of having "millions of dollars" in various banks, partly as an inheritance from his illustrious ancestor, partly as awards for his superlative academic achievements. This was not a man with Korsakoff's psychosis—he did not make preposterous confabulations—nor did he suffer from pseudologia fantastica, whose victims appear to believe their own stories and tell them to everyone who will listen. This man spoke in this vein only to the doctors and nurses (not to the other patients), who gave him small doses of neuroleptics until his malingering was confirmed. Meanwhile, he stopped parading his grandiose "psychosis," and it did not return after the medication was discontinued. He too was a patient whose correct diagnosis was malingering in an antisocial personality.

The forensic patient who held out the longest as a poseur with borderline personality disorder was a woman in her midtwenties who was transferred to a forensic hospital after an arrest for disorderly conduct—at a time when she appeared to be suffering from a profound disturbance of identity. Diagnosed originally as a "borderline patient with pseudologia fantastica; rule out paranoid schizophrenia," she presented a baffling clinical picture. Though she spoke unaccented American English, she claimed she was born in "Bohemia" and that her native tongue was "Bohemian." Seemingly unaware that the western part of Czechoslovakia had not used "Bohemia" as its official national name in many decades and had never called its language "Bohemian," she would, if asked to say a few sentences in Bohemian, rattle off a string of mumbled, nearly inaudible syllables. Unlike the man claiming to be the actor's great-great-grandson, this woman told the same Bunyanesque stories to everyone and appeared more often to believe what she was saying.

It was a matter of some two years on the forensic unit before she "came down to earth" and gave the staff some clue as to who she really was. As with the male patients described earlier, her goal also was to avoid prison. The dramatic, not to say theatrical, quality of this woman's self-presentation suggests a personality disorder made up chiefly of antisocial and *histrionic* elements rather than those of BPD. It was never clear whether her organizational level was truly borderline, since it seemed doubtful that she really believed she was a Bohemian-speaking native of Bohemia. If she did, she would have been psychotic. If not, she would have been (as eventually concluded) a sociopathic actress of such talent as to keep up her imposture for several years at a stretch.

FACTITIOUS ILLNESS

P. J. Resnick (1998) makes the cogent distinction that "factitious disorders involve the intentional production of symptoms in order to assume a patient role. The malingerer wants to *appear* sick, but the patient with factitious disorder wants to *be* sick, even when no one is watching" (p. 329).

Factitious illness is often referred to as Munchausen Syndrome[1] and often involves members of the medical profession, since they have the wherewithal to simulate disease (Stone 1977).

A nurse in her late twenties had been admitted to many hospitals, at first in the Boston area, where she then lived, for a baffling illness consisting of subcutaneous nodules about the abdomen and legs (anterior surface only). This was written up as a rare dermatologic disease with the eponymous name "Weber Christian panniculitis." During a hospitalization in New York, something about the peculiarity of the woman and the multiplicity of her hospitalizations made her intern suspicious. He discovered a cold-cream jar filled with a culture of staphylococcus aureus, hidden in her bedside radio, along with an array of needles—which she had been using, as it turned out, to give herself subcutaneous injections of those bacteria, by way of simulating Weber Christian disease. Once the deception was uncovered, the staff urged her to get psychiatric help and attempted to transfer her to the psychiatric wing. At this she flew into a rage and immediately signed out of the hospital. In retrospect, she had all the earmarks of borderline psychopathology (both as organization level and as BPD)—anger, self-destructiveness, stormy relations (with her family), and a severe disturbance of identity—though the term "borderline" was not widely used in that era.

The second case, also a nurse, was a patient at a prominent cancer center. This woman, also in her late twenties, was being worked up for a puzzling and profound anemia (hemoglobin of 3.5) that seemed both iron-deficient and hemolytic in character. A radioisotope study revealed a peculiarly jagged curve of red cell life. This "unbiological" curve aroused suspicions, and as with the first patient, a search was conducted when she was outside of her room. This led to the discovery of venipuncture paraphernalia: a garter belt for a tourniquet, a size 18 needle, and some tubing. With these items, she had been periodically dumping quantities of her own blood down the toilet. Con-

---

[1]There is an eerie symmetry to this erroneous appellation, for just as factitious illness is pretended illness, the Baron von Munchausen, an actual nobleman in the eighteenth century, was only the pretend-author of the fabulous tales and exploits allegedly emanating from his pen. The stories were written by an impoverished student, Rudolf Raspe, who (in the days when there was no copyright law) felt he could generate better sales if he ascribed his work to the much more well-known Baron von Munchausen.

frontation with the facts of her deception led to no better a result than with the first patient: she was furious about being found out and signed out against advice, refusing to be seen by a psychiatrist. Her psychopathology also involved borderline personality, but as with the first patient, the main condition was the antisociality: she used deceit to gain sympathy as an unfortunate victim of a severe anemia that the doctors, until they discovered her deception, could not figure out. She lived in a hostile interdependent relationship with her parents, had no social life, was acutely lonely, and chose this route to alleviate the frustration and barrenness of her life.

A third case concerned a divorced woman of twenty-six who had been admitted to an internal medicine ward because of a clotting disorder with widespread purpura (for a lengthier description, see Stone 1980, case 17). She had been a medical secretary with a broad knowledge of various diseases. Chronically embattled with her parents, whom she resented as controlling and selfish, she displayed boundless anger toward them and oscillated between cursing them out and spreading malicious rumors about them to neighbors—and playing on their sympathies by feigning Hodgkin's lymphoma, a cardiac condition necessitating a pacemaker, diabetes, and finally the purpuric condition. She "split" the hospital staff into two camps—a group that disliked her and another that felt sorry for her—and was hostile when they ultimately told her that her "purpuric condition" stemmed from the large quantities of aspirin she secretly had been swallowing to produce just this response. She was diagnosable as borderline with antisocial, narcissistic, and hysteric personality traits. For about three months after she left the hospital, she was treated by one of the authors (M.S.), but the treatment was a failure. She quit in a huff. As with borderline patients in whom antisociality outweighs the borderline aspects, therapeutic efforts often come to naught.

As we hope to have shown with the clinical examples in this chapter, treatment dilemmas in borderline patients may arise both from misdiagnosis, in the strict sense of the term, and from what one might better call "misemphasis"—the patient does show clinical signs and symptoms that meet BPD criteria but BPD is overshadowed by other clinical syndromes that require more urgent attention and have a more serious impact on prognosis. BPD is a common accompaniment of malingering and factitious illness, for example, but the latter two take precedence over the BPD in one's efforts to fashion an appropriate treatment strategy.

PART TWO
ADDRESSING THE
COMPLICATING FACTORS

CHAPTER 4

Sadomasochism

Sadomasochism in borderline patients is a reflection of internalized perse-cutory relationships between self and object representations; it is a common dynamic in this population, although its manifestations may be disguised or indirect. The sadomasochistic dynamic often dominates the transference, even early on in treatment. This can lead to dramatic self-destructive or sui-cidal acts choreographed in ways that enmesh the therapist, covert sadistic treatment of the therapist, which threatens to drive him away or invite un-conscious counteraggression. Such patterns can destroy the treatment before it gets off the ground, or they can produce chronic stalemates in which the patient and therapist are locked in a mutually painful embrace. This chapter examines the sources of sadomasochism in borderline patients and how it may best be dealt with in treatment. Sadomasochism is even more pervasive and intense at the more severe levels of personality pathology, particularly in the syndrome of malignant narcissism and in the antisocial personality; these are discussed in chapter 5.

The sadomasochistic dynamic provides the basic coloring not only of the patient's relation to the therapist but of the patient's experience of and be-havior toward himself. Relations both with the self (characterized by cut-ting, head-banging, and more subtle self-damaging and self-defeating patterns) and with others (finding ways to make others "squirm" or, alter-natively, provoking others to act in harsh, punitive ways) reflect the pa-tient's intensity and lack of integration of his self- and object-related aggression.

THE ROLE OF AGGRESSION
IN SADOMASOCHISM

A brief review of current thinking regarding the origin and vicissitudes of aggression may be helpful in understanding the development of sado-masochistic patterns (Kernberg 1992; Parens 1979). Factors contributing to the level of aggression in an individual include:

- Genetic and constitutional makeup: Biological studies have provided evidence of a relation between neurotransmitter function–the serotonergic and noradrenergic system in particular–and aggression (Siever 1993; Silk 1997)
- Developmental issues, especially early physical or emotional abandonment
- Severe early trauma and related chronic pain, where the early experience of pain induces aggressive responses: This includes psychological trauma, such as may even be imparted by a relentlessly teasing mother (Galenson 1986; Fraiberg 1983; Osofsky 1988)
- Chronic physical and/or sexual abuse or the witnessing thereof (Paris 1994)

The aggressive drive becomes internally structured as hatred in relation to an object. Hatred, often disguised in its surface presentation, develops as an attempt to eliminate pain by destroying the perceived bad object, which is experienced as willfully trying to kill, attack, destroy, annihilate, and control the self. In turn, the subject wants to take revenge, destroy, induce suffering in, or control the object. These elements of hatred are perpetuated as long as the split-off, internalized, hated object remains unintegrated and is repeatedly projected in the effort to control the perceived threat, and perhaps to gain vengeance.

Hatred does not always declare itself openly, especially since the individual who hates may be reluctant to acknowledge that feeling in herself. The internal object relation involving hate includes a persecutory object and the victim-self. As with all internalized relationship dyads, the patient identifies unconsciously with both the self representation and the object representation—the victimizer as well as the victim. The victimizer part may be relatively apparent in the patient's self-destructive behaviors and attitudes and behaviors toward the therapist, but it remains out of the patient's awareness.

Patients may enter treatment complaining of their weakness and fragility–a feeling that is real–but unaware of the power of their aggression as it is manifested in actions toward themselves, their therapists, and others in their lives. This is the "waif" whose distress and apparent helplessness stem not so much from simple weakness–which could make use of and respond to the help that is offered–as from the conflict between manifestations of the weak self, which may seek help, and the aggressive self, which may never express itself explicitly in words ("I hate you") but whose actions may continually attack and undermine the patient, the therapist, and the work they are attempting to do. Such cases are often referred out by therapists who lament that the poor, long-suffering patient cannot seem to get better when, in fact, the therapist cannot admit or even acknowledge that he feels beat up, abused, and threatened by the patient.

Aggression, rage, and hatred are, of course, not exclusively the province of borderline patients. The manifestation of these affects in the individual personality depends on both the level of aggression and the degree to which it is neutralized, encapsulated, projected, or integrated. Nonpathological manifestations include:

- Direct and not excessive expression of aggression in appropriate circumstances in an integrated personality
- Its fusion in sensual responses, which include the erotization of mild pain (for example, tickling)
- Integration of the primitive superego with a more modulated direction of aggression against the self in the form of self-criticism or exaggerated guilt feelings, and against the other in the form of "justified indignation," with a tendency to controlling, dominant, aggressive relations with others, rationalized on a "moral" basis
- Sublimation and creative use of aggression

Pathological manifestations of aggression involve the exaggeration of nonpathological manifestations:

- Exaggerated aggression in the sexual domain that may result in perversion or paraphilia while the rest of the personality proceeds along normal developmental lines
- Exaggerated aggression absorbed in the domain of the superego that can push the individual into a depressive-masochistic person-

ality (see chapter 8 for a discussion of the depressive-masochistic personality)

- When the excessive aggression is not absorbed into the domain of either sexuality or the superego, the types of characterological expressions of sadomasochism that are very common in borderline personality—self-mutilation, suicide attempts, aggression toward others, and generalized violent explosive behavior

ADDRESSING THE
SADOMASOCHISTIC TRANSFERENCE

In the psychotherapy of the borderline patient, hatred is frequently expressed in sadomasochistic transferences. The sadistic and masochistic roles can be exchanged back and forth, as will be seen in the clinical examples discussed here.

Patients display several typical forms of sadomasochistic transference: an arrogant attitude, characterized by grandiosity, curiosity, and pseudo-stupidity (Bion 1968); a view of the therapist as rejecting, destructive, and aggressive while it is the patient who actually acts in those ways; being self-accusatory and attacking.

The sadomasochistic personality may have paranoid traits but is not the same as the paranoid personality. In the latter, the aggression is more "successfully" projected and becomes enacted only if the projection meets with a "compliant target"—namely, someone easily provoked to become aggressive toward the patient. In the sadomasochistic personality, the enactment of suffering and victimization is much more pronounced and coincides with the paranoid projection of aggression.

Although the self-destructiveness of borderline patients is multidetermined (Yeomans, Hull, and Clarkin 1994; Simeon et al. 1992; Gardner and Gardner 1975), from a dynamic point of view it often represents the acting out of a sadomasochistic drama, which, if therapy goes well, becomes concentrated in the transference. The key to working through the sadomasochistic dynamics of a borderline patient is to be attentive to the roles enacted in the transference-countertransference. The therapist may find himself being induced to play the role of sadist, or masochist, or, most likely, to alternate between them. If the therapy is unfolding in the context of a clearly established treatment frame, the transference-countertransference paradigms may develop around a manifest content involving details of the treatment (scheduling of sessions, payment of fees, and so on) and/or through enactments within sessions. For example, a patient came to the therapist's waiting room when it was not time for her session and sat there loudly sobbing. In the next session, the patient explained this behavior by saying that she "just needed to be near" the therapist. On further exploration, it emerged that the patient was enraged at what she perceived as the therapist's indifference to her (therapist experienced as persecutor) and wanted to punish and humiliate him (patient acting as persecutor) by showing his other patients what harm he had done to her.

Therapy of the borderline patient with sadomasochistic trends requires certain preconditions:

- Drawing up a clear treatment contract
- Maintaining the boundaries of the therapy (boundaries ensure that aggression cannot be acted out beyond certain limits; if it exceeds these limits, it threatens or even destroys the possibility of the therapeutic endeavor)
- Being sensitive to and tolerant of sadistic and masochistic material, especially as it is manifested through the defense of projective identification (it is especially important that the therapist tolerate his or her countertransference aggression or masochism without acting it out)
- Gradually helping the patient to acknowledge his or her aggression, including the pleasurable aspects of it, and to realize that aggression is not necessarily negative
- Being "impatient" in the individual session (rather than absorbing the aggression) but patient over time, acknowledging that understanding and change take place slowly and that only active interpretive work in each session combined with the willingness to tolerate long-range, extended work will significantly modify this pattern in the transference
- Remaining aware that the patient could have a severe negative therapeutic reaction based on her internal expectation that she could be loved only by someone who physically abuses or batters her (a more severe type of negative therapeutic reaction than those based on envy or unconscious guilt)

The most challenging cases are often those in which the patient's superficial fragility veils the sadomasochistic dynamic. The patient comes in suffering. The therapist offers help. The patient appears to comply with the treatment but does not get better. In subtle ways, the patient, who might be characterized as a "help-rejecting complainer," rejects all the therapist's efforts. If the therapist does not have a formulation of the situation, he is at risk of acting out in the countertransference. A continued awareness of the internal world of the patient with sadomasochistic dynamics reminds the therapist that even a fragile-appearing patient may function in relation to persecutory/persecuted self and object representations. Within her psyche, the patient experiences on-going self-attack in terms of both punitive self-criticism and self-destructive acting out. Within the therapeutic setting, the patient both projects the aggressive object representation onto the therapist (therapist as sadist) and enacts that representation by finding ways to make the therapist worry, incriminate himself, or squirm (therapist as masochist). The potential countertransference dilemma involves the therapist's fear that not resolving the patient's desperate neediness and distress is sadistic, whereas in fact it is more likely a realistic limitation in face of the patient's primitive psychological functioning. Yet the therapist's fear of being depriving and sadistic can lead to a counterphobic giving in and yielding to unreasonable demands from the patient (for example, in relation to phone calls or medication), with the end result that the therapist assumes a masochistic position.

Basic aspects of the treatment arrangements may become the vehicle for transmitting a sense of mistreatment or persecution: ending sessions on time may be seen as an aggression; adhering to the exploratory psychodynamic method rather than providing encouragement or advice may be experienced as cruel deprivation; and so on. When the patient expresses these feelings overtly, the therapist is better able to observe and understand this part of the patient's inner world as it manifests itself in the negative transference, but the patient may not express such feelings, withholding them from the therapeutic dialogue. The latter situation is associated with a higher level of acting out and a higher risk of dropping out of treatment (see Yeomans et al. 1992).

The patient generally remains unaware of her enactments of the aggressive, sadistic role during the early phases of therapy. Uncomfortable with this self representation, the patient generally projects this aspect of her inner world, leading to a subjective experience of persecution with regard to the therapist.

CASE EXAMPLE

Illustrating many of these themes is the case of Ms. Q., a twenty-two-year-old woman who was referred for consultation to Dr. A. by another therapist, Dr. E., who had been treating her for three years and was frustrated after her fifth serious suicide attempt in that period of time. It soon became apparent that Dr. E. was interested in transferring the patient but had difficulty stating this explicitly.

Ms. Q.'s characteristic method of attempting suicide was to leave the apartment she shared with her boyfriend, check into a hotel, leave phone messages for her therapist and boyfriend, and take an overdose of serious proportions. When she awoke or was aroused from her sedated state, Ms. Q. would be taken to the hospital for medical treatment followed by a period of inpatient psychiatric treatment. In discussing her suicidality in the evaluation sessions with Dr. A., Ms. Q. "assured" him that she would be safe for a while because she had "got it out of her system" for the time being. She added that suicidal feelings would most certainly come back because they always did, suggesting that any therapeutic effort would make no difference since her attempts at self-destruction seemed to have a power and a life of their own.

Ms. Q. was the oldest of two daughters born to a middle-class southern family. Her parents, both professionals, were considered liberal and nonconformist within their community. The patient described a more disturbed side to their private behavior, which included cavorting around the house naked and inviting the patient to join in when she was nine or ten years old. She also described her father's alcoholism and sadistic behavior, such as killing the family's pet rabbits when they grew to be adults because they were no longer as cute to him as when they were young and because he did not want to be bothered with their mess. She added that on one occasion she almost killed a pet rabbit herself because of her belief that this would spare the animal a more painful death at her father's hands. Ms. Q.'s mother related to her as a confidante at an early age, engaging her daughter in discussions of her intimate relations and problems with the father.

Ms. Q. reported chronic suicidal ideation starting at age six. As an adolescent, she began to date married men twice her age, some of whom were friends of parents. She was gratified by her parents' reaction of shock and annoyance. Other behaviors that began in adolescence were drinking, restricting food, cutting and burning herself, and pulling out tufts of her hair. Ms. Q. entered therapy at age fourteen but was never open with that therapist because she viewed him as an agent of her parents. She herself sought out therapy in college because of recurrent depressed moods, drinking, and other self-destructive behaviors. She considered her therapist well intentioned but ineffectual.

After college, Ms. Q. moved in with an old boyfriend from high school. He was the son of a friend of her parents for whom she had had romantic feelings. Moving in with her boyfriend provided a brief respite from her depression and suicidal feelings, but they returned six months later. When Ms. Q. again sought out therapy, she felt it could not really help her change, but she hoped it would solve her loneliness. The three-year therapy was marked by a number of suicide attempts, as mentioned earlier. When Dr. E. was referring the case, he explained that he had had the role of the good father in her life and that Ms. Q. frequently expressed the wish to be adopted by him. At the same time, he experienced her as very controlling of him. She was sensitive to separations and "routinely" made a suicide gesture or attempt when he left on vacation. He felt he "could not take another suicide attempt," and he began to allow her to have weekly phone sessions when he was away. When Ms. Q. made a suicide attempt even after that arrangement was in place, Dr. E. decided to terminate the therapy. Yet he experienced ambivalence and guilt about his decision. Even though she "took up a lot of time" and he felt "a lot of responsibility for her," he believed she "had not been dealt a fair hand in life" and said he would consider taking her back into treatment.

Dr. A. began his work with Ms. Q. by obtaining an adequate history in order to establish his own diagnostic impression, formulation, and ideas for the treatment contract. Her active problems included recurrent suicidality, episodic drinking, a characterological sense of worthlessness and hopelessness, and lack of any structured activity–school or work–in spite of the fact that she appeared quite intelligent. In addition, Ms. Q. described intense erotic feelings for her previous therapist and the belief that she could not relinquish him even though they had stopped their work together. Her new therapist explained to Ms. Q. that his own work with her could proceed only if they agreed on a frame that would define the nature of their work and safeguard it as much as possible from the risk of derailment that followed from her wish that her therapist be actively involved in her life (for example, solving her problem of loneliness and gratifying her wish to feel special).

Ms. Q. initially said she did not like the tone of the therapy that Dr. A. was proposing because she felt she needed a therapy that provided more immediate support. She did not know how she could deal with the intensely dysphoric feelings she was subject to if she did not have a therapist who would provide her with direct and overt support and encouragement. Dr. A. explained that the best support he could offer her was to understand the depth and complexity of her inner world and to support her growth and change in a way that would preclude his supporting the continuation of her pathological patterns; he added that he could also help her find the kind of therapy she seemed more interested in. Ms. Q. then agreed to try to work with him, offering the view that it was like a "bitter pill" that she knew she needed.

In discussing the treatment contract, Dr. A. discussed how therapy would approach the particular behaviors that might threaten the exploratory therapy: drinking, restricting food, having no purposeful activity in her life, attempting suicide, and withholding information in session. Dr. A. explained the expectation that Ms. Q. would take responsibility for these behaviors and outlined the contingencies that would apply if these behaviors became active problems. For example, he told her that it would impair his ability to be available to her as a therapist interested in helping her understand herself if he became involved in the actions of her life, such as arranging for emergency services if she made a suicide attempt. Although discussion of her suicidal thoughts and fantasies was very relevant to their work together, it was her responsibility to seek appropriate intervention from family, friends, or emergency services if she considered herself at risk to act—or did act—in a suicidal way between sessions. Ms. Q. said she understood the rationale for these conditions, acknowledging that her suicidal behaviors had served, among other things, to punish her previous therapists for perceived wrongs and abandonments and to involve them in her life outside of therapy sessions. She agreed to begin therapy.

In the first session after they drew up the contract, Ms. Q. told Dr. A. that she had cried after the preceding session because she experienced him as a robot who had no feelings or concern for her. She believed too much was being asked of her and said the treatment contract created a situation in which she felt like he was asking her to "cross the abyss without a rope." She said that she needed someone to help her and that people expected too much of her, seeing her as healthier than she was. Dr. A. wondered as he listened to Ms. Q: *Am I indeed asking too much of her? Is she incapable of taking responsibility for her actions?* He had, of course, considered this in his initial evaluation of the patient. He had not judged her as generally unable to be responsible for her actions, although he was aware of both the potential for regression and the possibility that his evaluation was inaccurate. He went on to consider other possibilities. Was her presentation in this session the manifestation of a transference pattern, the weak child in relation to the unempathic, uninvolved, and uncaring parental figure? Or was the self representation relating to a more actively malevolent parental figure, one who saw and understood her distress but sadistically enjoyed the sight of her suffering ("over the abyss without a rope")? In the session, he attempted to help her see more clearly how she experienced the relationship with him; without denying the subjective reality of her experience, he implicitly reassured her that such things could be experienced and discussed in therapy without the need to either deny the meaning of the experience or act on the intensity of the feeling.

The next morning, Dr. A. checked his answering machine for messages at about 9:00 A.M., his usual practice. There were three messages relating to Ms. Q. The first was from her, and it was time-stamped at 10:00 P.M.; she stated that she was feeling suicidal and that, although she knew Dr. A. would not do anything about it, she thought it might be relevant for him to know. The second message was from the psychiatrist on call in the local emergency room; Ms. Q. was there, and he was hoping to get some information from Dr. A. The third call was from Ms. Q.'s boyfriend, who informed Dr. A. that she had been admitted to the inpatient psychiatric unit.

Dr. A. had a number of reactions to these messages. He wondered whether he had missed anything in the previous day's session. He asked himself whether he was right in recommending the relatively ungratifying experience of exploratory therapy for this patient. As he reflected more on the situation, he considered the night's events and the patient's phone message in terms of the treatment contract. She had maintained a fine line in calling him without involving him, strictly speaking: she had called him because she thought it "relevant" that he know about her suicidal feelings, not because she was asking him to intervene. She had in fact reported to the emergency room for evaluation, as she had agreed to do. One understanding of her call was as a test of his own commitment to the treatment contract. She had let him know that she was suicidal and did not say that she was planning to go to the emergency room. Did she want to see what he would do with this information? Did she want to determine whether the power of her suicidal ideation was stronger than the words of the treatment contract?

Dr. A. felt that, while Ms. Q. had nudged the frame established by the contract a bit, nothing in her behavior was outside the realm of what he might expect from a borderline patient in the induction phase of therapy; she had not, he concluded, acted in violation of their contract.

Dr. A. communicated with Ms. Q. and with the hospital psychiatrist treating her, confirming that when she was deemed stable she could return to outpatient treatment with him. Her suicidal ideation resolved quickly, and she was discharged after four days in the hospital. In the first post-hospital session, Ms. Q. began by asking Dr. A. why he treated borderline patients, since they "were awful and didn't get better." Dr. A. wondered whether her question and comment had anything to do with her recent hospitalization. She responded that she felt she had to go into the hospital to "get Dr. E. [her prior therapist] out of her head," since she was still preoccupied with erotic feelings for him. Dr. A. wondered whether the hospitalization was not, in fact, an attempt to retreat from becoming preoccupied with him (Dr. A.) now that they had just begun therapy. He did not focus on the suicidal ideation that had been the stated reason for Ms. Q.'s hospitalization. Instead, he pursued two hypotheses: that seeking hospitalization was a way of testing his commitment to the treatment contract, and that she might be starting to have strong feelings for him, including erotic feelings that she could discuss only as displaced onto Dr. E.

In the second post-hospital session, Ms. Q. mentioned the return of suicidal ideation but quickly shifted the topic to her feelings for Dr. E. by saying, "I'd like to take him with me." Dr. A. was less quick to suppose that this hatred and aggression applied to him than he had been in wondering whether she was displacing her erotic feelings for him onto Dr. E. Toward the end of the session, Ms. Q. asked whether she could be hospitalized for the duration of the therapy. Dr. A. took this as an expression of her ability to experience her dysphoric affects within the context of the session—a sign, he felt, that she had begun to be able to work within the frame of the treatment, even though it was difficult. He responded to her question by saying that he empathized with how difficult it was to truly work in therapy, but that long-term hospitalization was a thing of the past.

Dr. A.'s assessment that Ms. Q. had effected the transition into therapy with him was mildly shaken when he checked his messages two days later on a Saturday morning. The psychiatrist on call at the emergency room had tried to contact him at 1:00 A.M. to see whether he could help in the assessment of Ms. Q. She had been hospitalized again for suicidal ideation. Dr. A.

held to his hypothesis that this was part of a rocky induction into therapy. He reassured himself that she had acted in accord with the treatment contract and hoped this latest hospitalization was a sign that she was channeling her affects, albeit with some testing, into the frame of the treatment. Her suicidal ideation again cleared quickly, and she was discharged on the day of her next session with Dr. A.

She began that session by criticizing the hospital for the lack of safety there, explaining that she had broken a glass in her room and would have been able to cut herself since the staff did not notice. Dr. A. suggested that she might also be expressing a feeling that he had missed something and that she was not safe in treatment with him. She switched the topic to Dr. E., saying that working with him was unsafe because she had actually managed to get him to break boundaries in small ways–for example, answering her questions about his travels–and that, even though she had obtained what she ostensibly wanted from him, it made her nervous that she could draw him out of role. Dr. A. was reassured, taking these comments to mean that, in spite of her complaints that he was like a robot, she sensed that she was safer in therapy with someone who did not respond to her seductive appeal. He was curious about the suicidal ideation that had led once again to hospitalization, but Ms. Q. responded: "I didn't think you wanted to hear about that. I thought your contract kept that out of our work together." Dr. A. noted this distortion of his discussion of suicidality. He suggested to the patient that her hospitalizations, which she must have assumed had some impact on him, were an expression of the part of her that resented his emphasis on the boundaries that defined their work together. He suggested that she was experiencing a good deal of confusion–a hallmark of the early phase of therapy with borderline patients–in that on one level she knew the boundaries were essential, while on another level she experienced them as rejection and resented them. He went on to suggest that her two hospitalizations were an expression of her anger over the way he had set up the treatment.

Ms. Q. said there was no point in discussing her anger because she realized that Dr. A. was impervious to anything she might want to do to affect him. She went on to say there were more important things to discuss, such as her attempt to seduce one of the nurses at the hospital. Ms. Q., who was attracted to both men and women, had felt drawn to Dawn, a nurse on the psychiatric unit. She was frustrated that Dawn rejected her idea of meeting outside of the hospital, but she had managed to slip Dawn her phone number. Dr. A. took this as more evidence of a rapidly developing erotic transference and asked Ms. Q. whether she had thoughts or fantasies of meeting him outside of session. She responded that there would be no use to such fantasies because she knew he would not respond except to reject her. As the session ended, Dr. A. wondered what the next manifestation of her erotic feelings for him might be and how long it would take before Ms. Q. would be able to acknowledge and discuss these feelings in session.

In the next session, Ms. Q. began with the news that she had spoken to Dr. E. regarding some overdue insurance forms he had failed to send in. In discussing her phone conversation with him, she commented in a matter-of-fact way that "he gets scared very easily"; referring to the tone of anxiety she perceived in him when they spoke, she expressed surprise that he would respond to her that way. When Dr. A. asked whether she thought he himself might be afraid of her, she replied: "Are you kidding? You and your contract . . . that protects you from everything." She added that his lack of concern for her reminded her of her parents. She assumed he had seen "too many borderline patients" to be worried by her and likened his attitude to the callousness she had developed toward the homeless she walked over on the sidewalk. Dr. A. was about to pursue this perception of him when Ms. Q. interjected that she had actually received a phone call from the nurse at the hospital and that they had set up a meeting. Dr. A. was concerned about this acting out; although he was aware that it had to be directly related to feelings in the transference, he became preoccupied with the question of whether he should alert the hospital that a nurse appeared to be violating boundaries with a patient. The session ended with Dr. A. pondering this issue.

The day before the next session, Dr. A. received a phone message from a very distressed Ms. Q. The message stated that she knew she was not to call him except in cases of emergency, but she was in a state of panic and unsure of her safety because she had met with Dawn, who had proposed a murder-suicide pact. Dawn, who had been struck by Ms. Q.'s fascination with suicide, would torture and kill her and then kill herself. Dr. A. returned the call and established that, though shaken, Ms. Q. felt that she was not at risk and could plan to come to the next day's session without any further intervention in the meantime. The situation left Dr. A. more preoccupied than before with the question of whether to notify the hospital of the apparent rogue nurse on the staff. He had worked in a hospital himself for many years and could identify with the concerns of the hospital psychiatrist, who would want to know of the potential threat to the treatment milieu. On the other hand, he reflected on what his patient was doing in her interaction with him. She had succeeded in arousing acute concern in him and had brought him to the verge of taking action in a matter that regarded her directly. His training to focus on issues as they developed within the therapeutic field between the patient and himself caused him to refrain from taking immediate action and to reflect further on the situation. His ongoing conflict about how to proceed led him to call on a colleague for consultation.

Dr. A.'s colleague, Dr. M., listened to the case and suggested that Dr. A. was experiencing a blind spot with regard to the central role of the patient's sadism in all that had transpired in the treatment thus far. Dr. M. referred back to the initial phone message reporting suicidal ideation and Ms. Q.'s hospitalization soon after the treatment contract had been discussed. He felt that this was not merely a test of Dr. A.'s commitment to the contract but also a sadistic attack in response to her experience of him as indifferent to her. It was the putting into action of the angry and hostile part of the patient's response to the treatment contract and the "robotic" Dr. A. Ms. Q.'s second hospitalization, just when Dr. A. was telling himself that she was settling into treatment, was another attack on him.

When Dr. A. again seemed to take the actions of her life in stride, but without clearly and directly addressing her aggression and sadism, Ms. Q. increased the intensity of her sadistic response to him by involving the nurse in her drama. As long as the action was between the patient and Dr. A., he felt comfortable with it, even though this acceptance involved denying the full character and intensity of the action. When Ms. Q. engaged a third party in the situation–someone who was both out of the therapeutic field and yet partially within it by virtue of her status at the hospital with which Dr. A. was associated–he began to feel uncomfortable because the patient seemed to be playing Russian roulette, using another individual as the revolver, and possibly him as the target, since he now felt like the man who knew too much with regard to the hospital nurse.

When Ms. Q. arrived for her session the day after the call about the murder-suicide pact, Dr. A. was ready to hear all the details of that development. Instead, Ms. Q. began the session by reporting a dream. The dream, which included images of torture, was not unrelated to the theme of her enactment. Nonetheless, to follow up her phone call with the narration of a dream and no explicit mention of the murder-suicide pact seemed a further enactment of aggression to Dr. A. He was still in a quandary, however, as to how to proceed. His principles of therapy would have him address the themes and affects active in the transference and countertransference. Yet his concerns about real danger, both to Ms. Q. and to other patients coming in contact with the nurse, kept him from freely addressing the transference-counter-transference issues. The dilemma he experienced provides a good example of the need to separate the pressure of external situations from the work of the therapy, since that pressure can impair the therapist's ability to work effectively with the material presented to him.

Dr. A. attempted in this session to help Ms. Q. see the risk of the situation she had created, a situation that she now passed off as a momentarily scary, but in reality innocent, fantasy discussion with Dawn. Dr. A. was exasperated in the face of her minimization of the events that had led her to panic the day before. He also secretly hoped that if he said the right thing, she would proceed to do the right thing and take responsibility for notifying the hospital of Dawn's inappropriate behavior. When this idea came up, the patient expressed concern that she could ruin Dawn's career. Dr. A. took the opportunity to suggest that she was afraid of her own potential for aggression. Ms. Q. agreed, but without affect. Dr. A. failed to link her capacity for aggression with the way she was treating him. The session ended in frustration for Dr. A.

Dr. A. consulted again with his colleague, who felt that Dr. A. was falling into the common error of becoming so immersed in the patient's world that he was beginning to accept highly pathological material as almost normal. Dr. M. reminded him how common it is for therapists to experience a kind of brainwashing as they are repeatedly exposed to a particular pattern of pathological behavior. He encouraged Dr. A. to take a step back periodically and ask himself what relatively normal behavior would be under the circumstances evolving in the therapy. With the help of this outside perspective, Dr. A. reflected that his patient's response to the proposed murder-suicide pact did not fall within any normal range. He could imagine a normal individual calling the police for protection, alerting the hospital to the staff member's aberrant behavior, enlisting friends and family to help keep her safe, or, at the very least, cutting off contact with the threatening person immediately and permanently. Ms. Q., on the other hand, had gone from a state of panic to the position that Dawn's talk was innocent fantasy and that there was no reason to stop seeing her. Dr. M. suggested to Dr. A. that this would be a time to delineate fully the self representation at play behind Ms. Q.'s actions, especially since her actions were communicating much more forcefully than her words at this point, and he recommended that Dr. A. speak in terms that left no room for ambiguity.

Dr. A. agreed that he had been unconsciously shying away from the full impact of what Ms. Q. was bringing to him. He realized that her veil of ironic wit and sophisticated banter was covering a potentially lethal sadism that threatened both herself and him. She was reporting, and then undercutting the report, that she was going out with a potential murderer. Continuing this relationship revealed that the murderer in herself was active in the situation. If, as she then claimed, the talk of murder-suicide was nothing more than fantasy material, she was choosing a very risky way to test whether Dr. A. cared about her life. She was challenging him to care about her life in a way that revealed her own lack of caring about it.

Ms. Q. began the next session by referring again to her former therapist, saying that a brief glimpse of him on the sidewalk had provoked her to call Dawn to talk about the murder-suicide "fantasy." Dr. A. chose to intervene at this point more directly than he had before, stating: "There's a killer on the loose here." Ms. Q. responded with her typical irony: "What am I supposed to do? I can't plan it with you." Dr. A. was more aware now of his tendency to go along with this defensive irony and assumed that Ms. Q. had picked up on the fact that he shared a somewhat cynical sense of humor. Encouraged by his consultation with Dr. M., he avoided the temptation to back away from the material and pointed to her response as more evidence of what he was saying, that life and death issues were in play and that she increased the risk by creating a dangerous situation and then responding as though nothing were going on. It was like a game of "dare" in which the point is to see who will be the first to become concerned, or, conversely, who can maintain cool indifference the longest under increasingly threatening circumstances.

When Dr. A. did not back away from discussing the "killer part" of her that seemed to subtend what she was doing with Dawn and with him, Ms. Q. responded: "I think it's pointless then. I don't think I can do this therapy." Dr. A. heard this as both an attack—a rejection of the help he offered—and a sincere statement of her despair that she might not be able to deal with the intensity of affects that underlay her symptoms. His response was supportive in the way that expressive therapy is supportive: he communicated, both through his words and his attitude, his belief that the therapy welcomed and could deal with her most intense affects, fears, and fantasies.

After this session, Ms. Q. experienced some sleepless nights and came into session less perfectly put together than she previously had. She sobbed when she brought up her belief that she could never have children–a belief she had referred to earlier in the therapy with her characteristic ironic non-chalance–because of her fear that she would harm them. This material led back to discussion of the killer part in her and the need to acknowledge it, get to know it, and gain control of it so that it no longer wildly influenced her behavior. Ms. Q. realized that she had to break off her relationship with the nurse, and, furthermore, that she needed to report the nurse's behavior to the hospital head nurse.

Ms. Q's therapy continued long beyond the initial two months described in this case history. Her sadomasochism continued to manifest itself period-ically in her actions. However, after these key sessions, which led to the clear and direct naming of the killer in her, that part of her became an accepted el-ement of the therapeutic dialogue. It was no longer split off from her dis-course and isolated in her actions. The work of therapy could proceed with the sense of immediate risk and danger to all involved greatly reduced.

This vignette illustrates two main points. First, therapists are reluctant to acknowledge and accept the full extent of sadistic and masochistic elements in their patients. This reluctance stems from two sources: the discordance of this view of the patient with the image that she usually presents of herself, and the therapist's hesitancy to experience the full extent of his own reaction to such a patient. This hesitancy is related both to the fear that can be elicited in the therapist by full awareness of the patient's capacity for aggression and to the difficulty that therapists have accepting the extent of their own inner aggression, which is catalyzed by the interaction with such patients.

Second, this case illustrates the usefulness of direct interventions based on the method of delineating the self and other representations that subtend the patient's interactions, and the impact that such interventions can have in redirecting the course of the patient's behavior and the therapeutic dialogue. After the interventions described here, Ms. Q. was able to confront the sado-masochistic aspects of her inner world and her personal history without fleeing into the ironic glibness and detachment that had previously been her escape.

CHAPTER 5

Narcissism and Psychopathy

Severe forms of narcissistic pathology in borderline patients pose special difficulties for their treatment with psychodynamic psychotherapy. Narcissistic disorders may be conceptualized along a continuum based on the degree of superego pathology, the intensity of projective defenses, and the presence of ego-syntonic aggression. *Antisocial personality disorder,* marked by the preeminence of hatred in internalized object relations, the need to destroy good objects out of intense envy, and the absence of any internal set of values, stands at the most severe end of the spectrum. The *syndrome of malignant narcissism,* characterized by the ability to maintain some idealized object representations protected from the need to destroy and by the capacity for loyalty, has a somewhat better prognosis, although strong paranoid trends and ego-syntonic aggression remain factors to contend with. Finally, in *narcissistic personality disorder* there is a capacity to recognize good in others, albeit subject to envious attack, and to maintain an internalized value system. Here the prognosis is more positive, but the treatment must address the strong challenges posed by the narcissistic transference and countertransference. This chapter addresses the treatment of patients with psychopathy and severe forms of narcissism within the framework of transference-focused psychotherapy. We begin with a review of the psychodynamic structures underlying the psychopathic personality.

THE PSYCHODYNAMICS OF THE
NARCISSISTIC-ANTISOCIAL SPECTRUM DISORDERS

A contemporary psychoanalytic approach to the etiology of the antisocial personality disorder focuses particularly on the pathological intrapsychic structures of these patients, with a clear understanding that the psychic structure develops from the interaction between the earliest object relations, on the one hand, and the genetic and constitutionally given activation of affect dispositions, on the other; in other words, the pathology of early affect development and the pathology of early object relations interact from birth on. This contemporary psychoanalytic view integrates several factors: biological predispositions to excessive aggression derived from excessive activation of aggressive affects; the influence of early trauma in inducing aggressive affect, mediated by intense and prolonged pain; and the distortion of internalized object relations under the impact of severely pathological interactions in infancy and early childhood. Entering into this equation are abnormalities in the neurochemical systems that codetermine affect activation, deficits in early perceptive and cognitive functions derived from central nervous system pathology, such as those described in chapter 2, as well as the direct influence of severe distortions in early attachment derived from the experience of physical pain, physical and sexual abuse, or early abandonment. The more complex interaction between the infant and the parental figures, which determines the internalization of moral codes, plays a role as well.

We may now formulate, from a psychodynamic viewpoint, the characteristic psychic structural aspects of patients with antisocial personality disorder, as well as those of patients along the entire spectrum of narcissistic pathology with associated antisocial behavior. For our definition of the antisocial personality disorder we rely on the work of Robert Hare (1993) and Otto Kernberg (1992)—who reestablished the direct connection with Harvey Cleckley's (1941) classical description—and avoid the dilution of the concept that has occurred as a consequence of the *DSM* system.

The essential structural characteristic of the antisocial personality disorder proper is a severe absence or deterioration of the entire superego system. This means, in practice, that the earliest layer of superego precursors— namely, primitive, persecutory, aversive representations of significant others (onto whom primitive aggressive impulses have been projected)—dominates early experience, to the extent of excluding any internalization of the idealized, all-good, demanding, yet gratifying representations of significant others that normally constitute the second layer of superego precursors, or the early ego ideal. This second layer would normally neutralize the first layer of persecutory superego precursors. The virtual or total absence of such idealized object representations of the ego ideal precludes the normal toning down of fantasied threatening prohibitions and punishments from the first superego layer. Unable to mitigate these internal dangers, the individual is left with little recourse but to project them, leading to the perception of intense threats arising from the environment. As a consequence, the more advanced and realistic demands and prohibitions of the third level of superego precursors, corresponding to the advanced oedipal stage, cannot take shape and are experienced in a highly distorted way under the impact of projected aggression.

The resulting absence in the individual of a normally integrated superego—that is, of a system of internalized ethical and moral demands—brings about a total dependency on immediate external cues for the regulation of interpersonal behavior and a total lack of the normal support that superego functions provide to the individual's self-experience and identity formation. Only immediate admiration from others or indications of triumph and dominance over the external world provide a sense of security and self-esteem. The individual lacks any capacity for ethical self-regulation and empathy for others (with a moral and ethical dimension) as a significant motivational system in interpersonal relations. By means of projective mechanisms, the selfish, suspicious, combative attitude of a self deprived of superego regulation is attributed to all others, precluding the capacity for trust, intimacy, dependency, and gratification by the experience of love from others. The overall structural characteristics of these individuals, in summary, include the absence of a functioning, integrated superego and the hypertrophy of a threatened, endangered, violent self geared to face an essentially dangerous, violent world. This pathological, grandiose, aggressively infiltrated self is the most primitive type of "identification with the aggressor."

We can translate this overall structural system into the language of an internal world of unconscious fantasies that reflect this pathology of internalized object relations: thus, the world of the antisocial personality disorder is characterized by a basic experience of savage aggression from the parental objects; this world of violence is experienced as a constant background to all interpersonal interactions. The lack of any good, reliable object relationship transforms the longing for a good object relation into the sense that the good are weak and unreliable; a reaction of rage and hatred because of the frustrations derived from them; unconscious envy of the good objects because they act as if they were not dominated by a world of internal violence; and, as a defense against envy and resentment, a pathological grandiose self characterized by devaluation and contempt. Only the powerful matter in the external world, and they must be controlled, submitted to, manipulated, and, above all, feared, because the powerful are sadistic and unpredictable.

The transformation of pain into rage, and chronic rage into hatred, is a central affective development of these patients. The structural characteristics of hatred imply the relationship between an endangered self and a hateful and hated object that needs to be controlled, made to suffer in revenge, and ultimately destroyed. The projection of hatred brings about a basic paranoid orientation toward a hatefully perceived world, and psychopathic dishonesty, treacherousness, and aggression may be considered as essential defenses against that basic, paranoid stance. Given the facts that there are no standards of behavior other than crude self-interest and that the effects of impulsive rage and hatred determine the unpredictability of the aggressive behavior of powerful others, the need for cautious submission and evasion, a consistent manipulation of assumed aggressors, prevents the assessment and internalization of any value system.

In other words, the basic paranoid orientation of the antisocial individual and the psychopathic defenses against it interfere with any possible internalization of value systems, even the idealization of the value systems of the potential aggressor. In this regard, the antisocial personality proper is different from the syndrome of malignant narcissism, in which, in contrast, there is at least some idealization of the value systems of the powerful, an idealization of the pathological grandiose self in terms of self-righteous aggression, and the capacity for some identification with other powerful idealized figures as part of a cohesive "gang" that permits at least some loyalty and good object relations to be internalized. For the psychopath, in contrast, only power itself is reliable, and the pleasure of sadistic control is the major motivation system in a world clearly divided between the all-powerful and the despicable weak.

The differentiation that Henderson made between passive and aggressive psychopaths (Henderson 1939; Henderson and Gillespie 1969) is of significant clinical value. To begin with, the passive type is much less dangerous and therefore provides some potential "space" for a psychotherapeutic inter-

vention, questionable as its effectiveness may be. The eminent dangerousness of the violent psychopath, in contrast, makes the need for immediate
protection of the family and of society the highest priority in dealing with
these patients. The passive type of psychopath has been able to learn to deal
with the powerful by pseudo-submission and by outsmarting them, a passive-parasitic exploitiveness that at least implies the capacity to control immediate anger and rage and to transform it into the slow-motion aggression
of a "wolf in sheep's clothes." These patients can deny their own aggression;
in their cases, the division of the world into wolves and sheep is comple-
mented by the adaptive function of the wolf disguised among the sheep.

Regardless of the predominantly aggressive or passive character of the
antisocial personality, what is remarkable also is that gratification for such
individuals is still linked to bodily functions, to eating, drinking, drugs, and
alcohol; sexuality, divested of its object relations implications, is lacking in
love and tenderness. For the most severely aggressive psychopaths, sexual
sadism may become an invitation to murder, making these individuals extremely dangerous. Alternatively, to the extent that even the early sensual-
ity of bodily contact and skin eroticism is eliminated so that all capacity for
sexual gratification is globally extinguished, the dominance of this early aggression makes such individuals prone to replace sexual interaction with
senseless physical destructiveness, self-mutilation, and murder.

In the syndrome of malignant narcissism, the process by which the earliest aggressive superego precursors are either projected or internalized in the
form of a violent, grandiose, pathological self is modified by the capacity to
internalize at least some idealized superego precursors as well. Here the admiration of the powerful is matched by the capacity to depend on sadistic
and powerful but reliable parental images. The internalization into the self of
aggressive and persecutory as well as idealized superego precursors brings
about the more ordinary pathological grandiose self of the narcissistic personality, with the particular characteristic of the internalization of aggression
into this pathological grandiose self. The idealization of the powerful self
goes hand in hand with the capacity for some loyalty and a certain tolerance
of the third-level realistic superego demands and prohibitions. What obtains
is the typical syndrome of malignant narcissism: a narcissistic personality
with severe antisocial behavior, ego-syntonic aggression, and strong paranoid traits.

The next step in this continuum is the narcissistic personality proper, in
which a certain degree of superego development—with internalization of

the third level of more realistic demands and prohibitions—has evolved, while the pathological grandiose self constitutes, by its idealized nature, a massive defense against the awareness of unconscious aggression, particularly in its form of primitive, dominant envy. In fact, the defenses against unconscious envy represent the dominant dynamics of the narcissistic personality and, by the same token, signal the capacity of these individuals to recognize the good aspects of others that are envied and that they would want to incorporate. Here the antisocial behavior reflects the ego-syntonic, rationalized entitlement and greed of a pathological grandiose self, and conflicts between areas of superego deterioration and remnants of internalized value systems may evolve.

A basic question remains unanswered: Once a malignant intrapsychic structure has evolved—that is, a pathological grandiose self infiltrated with aggression dominates psychic functioning in the absence of the moderating and maturing reliance on an integrated superego—can psychosocial influences, and particularly psychotherapeutic treatment, be of any help? One aspect of this question relates to social influences that may facilitate antisocial behavior; the Milgram (1963) experiments in the United States and Zinoviev's (1984) analysis of socialized dishonesty as a major cultural characteristic of the totalitarian system of the former Soviet Union have made us dramatically aware of the power of these influences. Edith Jacobson (1971) has pointed to the "paranoid urge to betray" that is a part of paranoid structures in general, and Otto Kernberg (1998) has applied this analysis to the psychopathic regression of leaders in organizations that present a very high level of paranoiagenesis.

Are there healing influences that, either in early childhood or perhaps even in later years, may alter the psychopathic structure? We do have good evidence that the narcissistic personality with antisocial features may be effectively treated, and that even the syndrome of malignant narcissism is treatable. So far, to our knowledge, this has not yet been demonstrated for the antisocial personality proper. What complicates the question of prognosis is that, in many studies, the selection of individuals with antisocial behavior does not differentiate sharply between the antisocial personality proper and the less severe syndromes in which antisocial behavior dominates. We believe that it is absolutely crucial that sharp diagnostic differentiations in this field be reintroduced as a precondition for the evaluation of the effectiveness of various treatment modalities.

In what follows, we explore some guiding principles for the clinical management of patients with severe antisocial behavior based on the diagnostic considerations just discussed and on our clinical experiences in the Borderline Research Group at the Westchester Division of the New York Hospital–Cornell Medical Center.

THERAPEUTIC STRATEGIES AND TACTICS

In clinical practice, the spectrum of personality disorders ranging from the narcissistic personality with antisocial features, to the syndrome of malignant narcissism, to the antisocial personality proper (in both its passive-parasitic and aggressive forms) also presents with a significant degree of paranoid features. Insofar as the combination of antisocial behavior and primitive defensive mechanisms implies a projection of these antisocial tendencies onto others, the fear of being found out, mistreated, manipulated, or exploited is a frequent correlate of antisocial behavior. In fact, from a diagnostic, prognostic, and therapeutic viewpoint, it is always crucial, in all these cases, to evaluate jointly:

- The presence or absence of pathological narcissism—that is, of a narcissistic personality disorder
- The extent to which superego pathology dominates—that is, where the patient falls in the continuum of personality disorders, from the narcissistic to the antisocial personality
- The intensity of ego-syntonic aggression, whether directed toward the self (in the form of suicidal, parasuicidal, and/or self-mutilating and self-destructive behavior) or toward others (in the form of physical violence, homicidal tendencies, or a life-endangering, sadistic perversion)
- The severity of paranoid trends
- The stability of reality testing

The careful assessment of the patient's narcissistic features, antisocial behavior, superego integration, paranoid trends, severity and direction of aggression, and reality testing permits the clinician to determine the extent to which the patient can be relied on to communicate honestly, the dangerousness of the patient to himself and others—including the therapist—and the overall prognosis for the patient's capacity to sustain a psychotherapeutic relationship, as opposed to the likelihood of early dropout from treatment. The most general prognostic psychotherapeutic rule—namely, that the degree of antisocial tendencies and the quality of object relations determine the prognosis for any psychotherapeutic treatment—thus becomes much more specific and immediately useful for the therapeutic planning of this particular spectrum of patients.

ANTISOCIAL PERSONALITY DISORDER PROPER

What follows are psychotherapeutic strategies that derive directly from the criteria outlined here and thus depend on a careful, detailed, comprehensive diagnostic evaluation. The most urgent question in any patient who presents with severe aggressive or self-aggressive behavior is the extent to which there is a risk to the patient's life or to the lives of other persons, including the therapist. If the diagnosis is that of an antisocial personality disorder in the restricted sense (that is, following the criteria proposed by us and in harmony with Robert Hare's research, as contrasted to the looser set of criteria of *DSM-III* and *DSM-IV*), it is crucial to take protective measures involving the patient's family, social services, and, if circumstances warrant, the law in order to protect human life.

The prognosis for psychotherapeutic treatment under such circumstances is practically zero, and the main therapeutic task is to protect the patient, the family, and society from threatening aggressive behavior, including criminal behavior. When such patients possess dangerous weapons, the therapist must arrange immediately to have the weapons taken away from them. For example, one patient who consulted because of severe hypochondriacal symptoms turned out to be involved in the homosexual seduction of men whom he would lure into a hotel in the center city and then rob at gunpoint. The therapist formulated the categorical demand that the patient deliver his weapon before any further psychotherapeutic contacts as the first step in the patient's assessment; the therapist also consulted with his lawyer about his legal responsibilities in the case.

If the patient fulfills the criteria of an antisocial personality in a strict sense, but with aggressive or exploitive behaviors that do not immediately threaten physical harm to the patient or anybody else, the most urgent question is to ascertain the reason for the consultation. Is the family searching for help? Is the patient seeking protection from impending legal actions brought against him? Is the legal system trying to assess the patient's responsibility for criminal action? Have the family or social agencies pressed for the consultation as part of an effort to deal with the threats the patient represents for his environment? Is the patient being seen during a period of genuine psychotic regression? There does exist a small group of patients who constitute what traditional German psychiatry denominated pseudo-psychopathic schizophrenia, that is, patients who alternate between periods of extended psychotic illness that conform to the criteria for chronic schizophrenia and periods of either spontaneous development or medication-facilitated recovery of reality testing, at which time the patient fulfills all the criteria for an antisocial personality disorder. These patients constitute prognostically the most ominous group within the category of antisocial personality disorders and usually can be managed only under conditions of practically permanent reclusion in specialized psychiatric hospitals or psychiatric prison systems.

If the patient presents a passive or aggressive type of an antisocial personality disorder that does not immediately threaten physical harm to self or others, the first task, once the diagnosis has been established, is to protect the patient's family and the social environment from the long-term dangers derived from the patient's behavior. For patients with antisocial personality disorder who chronically steal from or exploit their families, are chronically violent without actual threat to life, or are chronically engaged in behavior that threatens to involve them with the law, such protective intervention may include psychotherapeutic consultations with the family or social agencies and law enforcement agencies. It is essential, of course, that psychotherapeutic contacts not be exploited as a protection against legal procedures, that the psychotherapist take all measures to ensure his own safety as a precondition for such interventions with the family, and that the therapist obtain specific information regarding his legal responsibilities.

Given the ominous prognosis for all psychotherapeutic treatments of these patients, it is the psychotherapist's responsibility, if and when he intends at all to begin psychotherapeutic work with a patient presenting this diagnosis, to make it an essential and strict precondition for the treatment to proceed that the patient discontinue the antisocial activity that is potentially threatening to himself or others. For example, a patient with a pedophilic perversion who is HIV positive would have to commit himself to absolute abstention from any pedophilic activity as a precondition for treatment. It would be absurd, of course, even to propose such a precondition to a patient who has not proven honest in his communication about his behavior.

One patient with chronic antisocial behavior, chronic suicidal tendencies, and self-mutilating behavior threatened to act on the impulse to cut herself with razor blades in the presence of the psychotherapist; she arrived at a later session with razor blades in her purse, now threatening to cut the therapist if she attempted to interfere with the patient's self-mutilating behavior. Before she could make a definite diagnosis regarding this patient's antisocial behavior, the therapist was appropriately motivated by this development to take immediate action to ensure her own safety: she refused to see the patient alone in a closed room and arranged for the patient's immediate hospitalization. Another patient, with the diagnosis of a passive type of antisocial personality disorder, had sequestered the money to be paid for taxes on his wife's business over several years, an act that led to the bankruptcy of the business once the Internal Revenue Service uncovered this fact. He wanted to enter psychotherapeutic treatment as a way to demonstrate to his wife his commitment to changing his behavior in order to avoid a separation and divorce. In the course of the evaluation of his psychopathology, in which the entire family was involved, it emerged that his wife was willing to give him another chance only under the condition of a total separation of their financial activities, thus precluding his continued economic dependency on her and forcing him to engage in productive work commensurate with his professional background. Psychotherapy was proposed to him under the condition that he would be responsible for the payment of his treatment based on his own work, with the understanding that the therapist's ongoing communication with the patient's wife and other family members would be an essential aspect of a long-range psychotherapeutic arrangement. Once it became clear to the patient that his psychotherapeutic treatment would no longer satisfy his wish to remain financially dependent on his wife and her family, he abruptly discontinued it.

Psychotherapeutic treatment with nondangerous antisocial personality disorders requires open communication with the patient and the entire family regarding the severity of the condition, the poor nature of the prognosis, and the need to maintain such open communication with the entire family in order to monitor the patient's compliance with the treatment conditions that all antisocial behavior be suspended. Psychotherapy also requires a realistic assessment and control of the patient's potential aggression toward self and others, and elimination of all secondary gains for the patient in entering psychotherapeutic treatment.

If a patient with an antisocial personality disorder presents with chronic lying as a major symptom, and the treatment conditions can be achieved—for example, in the case of an adolescent patient still living with and potentially under the control of the parents—the treatment arrangements should also include educational contacts with the family that stress the fact that nothing the patient says can be believed at face value and that the only reliable source of information is the patient's behavior. Therefore, the family has to make it very clear to the patient that his behavior, not any of his statements, will determine the nature of their interactions with him and the rights and privileges he will be granted in the home. If the adolescent steals consistently from the home, for example, to obtain funds for drug dealing or other activities, it may be a treatment condition, for the protection of the family, that such a youngster may no longer remain in the home and that institutional or foster care placement is the only alternative if stealing cannot be totally eliminated.

If the problem is lying rather than stealing, parental control may be much easier, and in the psychotherapeutic sessions, as long as the antisocial behavior is controlled in the external environment, the patient's chronic lying may be taken up as the dominant or unique transferential development until it is either resolved or demonstrated to be impossible to resolve. Nevertheless, in the case of patients with severely aggressive—rather than passive-exploitive—behavior, the rigorous control of that behavior represents an indispensable precondition for a psychotherapeutic treatment to proceed.

MALIGNANT NARCISSISM

When the diagnostic assessment is that of the syndrome of malignant narcissism rather than an antisocial personality proper—that is, the typical combination of a narcissistic personality structure, severe antisocial behavior, paranoid trends, and ego-syntonic aggressions directed against self and/or others—the prognosis improves and a particular psychotherapeutic strategy may be effective. Again, however, preconditions for the treatment include strict control of the antisocial behavior and of self- or other-directed aggression; development of a treatment structure that includes open communication regarding the patient's behavior outside the therapy hours with the family and the social system; elimination of all secondary gain of treatment for the patient; and the physical, social, and legal protection of the therapist.

In our experience, most of these patients require an initial period of hospital treatment to set up these treatment arrangements. When long-term inpatient treatment is available, psychodynamic psychotherapy may start on an inpatient basis, to be continued on an outpatient basis once the patient is ready to take on the responsibility for fulfilling the preconditions for treatment as part of her own treatment contract. Sometimes, however, outpatient treatment may be attempted from the beginning and an ordinary psychotherapeutic treatment contract may be set up. For example, one adolescent patient had severe behavior problems at school and committed acts of inordinate physical violence against other students and teachers, dealt drugs, had been cheating at school and lying to family members for some time, engaged in alcohol and drug abuse and sexual promiscuity, and had a leading position in a street gang. Although he presented a typical narcissistic personality structure, ego-syntonic aggression, severe paranoid traits, and antisocial behavior, he could maintain loyalty to his gang and to individual members, exhibit a nonexploitive dependency on some family members, and show authentic guilt feelings when a violent outburst produced a significant physical lesion in another boy. The establishment of a tight social control system, involving a psychiatric social worker who maintained ongoing contacts with the patient's family, school, and the local police regarding his gang-related activities, and strict control regarding his finances and whereabouts provided an adequate structure to attempt an outpatient psychotherapeutic relationship.

This patient began attending psychotherapeutic sessions only under the threats of his family to cut off all financial support unless he regularly did so. To undercut the development of magical or unrealistic expectations, the therapist made it very clear to the patient and his family that, although he was willing to undertake such a treatment, he was not very hopeful about a successful outcome. In the sessions, the patient alternated between berating the therapist as the agent of his parents and filling the hours with trivialities, while the therapist systematically focused on his deceptiveness in his relationship with the therapist and the functions of this deceptiveness in the therapeutic interaction. The therapist's analysis of the patient's perception of him as a corrupt agent of the parents, a foolish dispenser of quackery, and a dangerous enemy who was attempting to control his life while pretending to be on his side gradually helped the therapist to clarify the patient's projection of the characteristics of his own pathological, grandiose self onto the therapist. This analysis shifted the transference of the patient's profound conviction that in a world where everybody was everybody else's enemy only the powerful and the "wolves disguised as sheep" could triumph over the "suckers" who were their victims, from a typically psychopathic conviction into a paranoid one. In general, if and when a solid and unbreakable treatment frame can be established that provides space for the systematic analysis of the antisocial psychopathology expressed as psychopathic transference, that analysis may gradually resolve the psychopathic transference and transform it into a predominantly paranoid transference. The paranoid transference may subsequently be explored, as it is with the severe paranoid regressions that develop in non-antisocial narcissistic personalities and in patients with borderline personality organization (see chapter 7).

With a patient who is able to communicate honestly about his external life, the therapist can use that information about behavioral problems outside the sessions, as well as the development of severely regressive behaviors in the sessions, to transform interpretively the patient's pathological behaviors into cognitive and affective experiences in the transference, which can be explored and worked through. With a patient whose chronic deceptiveness prevents the therapist from accurately assessing pathological behaviors outside the sessions, the therapist must have a reliable network of information about the patient that permits the therapist to bring the pathological behavior expressed in the patient's life into the sessions. For this patient, as well as for all patients with severe acting-out tendencies, the transformation of what amounts to automatic, repetitive behavior patterns into affectively invested fantasies in the transference is a major task during extended periods of the treatment.

Whether the therapist relies on the patient's communication regarding his life outside the sessions and his behavior during the sessions, or whether the therapist utilizes additional information from other sources, the general principles of transference-focused psychotherapy can determine the issue on which to focus in the treatment hours. As a general psychotherapeutic priority, the therapist should always first consider whether interventions are urgently needed to forestall threats of danger to self and others, disruption of the treatment, dishonesty in the communication, acting out outside and inside the sessions, and trivialization of the communication. Second, it is essential to focus on the material that affectively pre-dominates in the total patient material, including the patient's verbal com-munication, his nonverbal behavior, and the countertransference. During extended periods of time in the treatment of these patients, whose commu-nication of their subjective experience is such a relatively "weak channel," careful evaluation of the patient's behavior and the therapist's countertrans-ference usually provides the most important cues to what is affectively dom-inant and needs to be explored.

This brings us to the problems in the countertransference in the treatment of patients with severely antisocial behavior. It is important, to begin with, that the therapist find some potentially likable, human aspect of the patient, an area of ego growth that could constitute the initially minimal yet essen-tial base for authentic communication from the therapist to the patient. In other words, the therapist's position of technical neutrality implies a gen-uine commitment to finding what he expects, or hopes, will constitute a still available core of object relation investment, of ordinary humanity, within the patient; within this core resides the capacity for authentic dependency and the establishment of a therapeutic relationship.

The therapist's comments start from an implicit alliance between the ther-apist in role and that preserved core aspect of the patient's personality, in contrast to the therapist's consistent confrontation of those aspects of the pa-tient's internal life identified with the primitive, sadistic, corrupt, antisocial, death-desiring parts of his personality. These patients' internal world of ob-ject relations is populated by primitive, sadistic representations of self and others and their interactions with masochistic, devalued, threatening, or cor-rupt enemies. At the beginning, the therapist may only be able to assume the existence of a somewhat normal self representation in the middle of this nightmarish world, but this assumption permits the therapist systematically to confront the patient's imprisonment in this world without equating such interpretations with an attack on the patient.

This means that, in spite of the patient's projection of his primitive super-ego precursors onto the therapist and the consequent perception of any crit-ical comment from the therapist as a savage attack to be fended off, it is important that the therapist firmly maintain a moral stance without becom-ing moralistic, and a critical attitude without letting himself be seduced into an identification with projected sadistic images; nor should the therapist be tempted into a defensively seductive, mutually manipulative style of communication that reinforces the denial of the severe aggression rooted in the patient's internal world.

Through provocative behavior, the patient will attempt to move the therapist out of that position of technical neutrality and authentic human concern and either into the role of a sadistic persecutor of the patient, the patient's masochistic victim, or a manipulative, essentially indifferent authority, or into a total emotional withdrawal from the patient. Paradoxically, a therapist's pseudo-investment—a friendly surface that denies the aggression in the countertransference or reflects a basic indifference toward the patient—may bring about an apparent "warming up" of the therapeutic relationship without a resolution of the underlying dishonesty in the patient's communication. More fundamentally, such pseudo-investment also makes it impossible to resolve the severe denial and splitting processes defending against the aggressive implication of the patient's antisocial behavior.

The protection of an honest investment on the therapist's part requires the objective safety of the therapist. Whenever the therapist feels threatened by the patient's pathology or by the patient himself, the first step has to be for the therapist to ensure his own physical, emotional, social, and legal safety. That safety must take precedence over any other consideration, because it is the very precondition for an authentic investment in the psychotherapeutic endeavor, and therefore a basic guarantee for the survival of the therapy.

The investment described here precludes the therapist's "going out of his way" to try to help an impossible patient; it requires that he maintain at all times a realistic boundary to his investment. In contrast, the therapist who, with the messianic attitude that impossible cases can be helped and saved, goes overboard to provide such patients with a "corrective emotional experience" of total dedication in the face of their provocative behavior courts the risk of his own denial of the negative aspects of the countertransference—the gradual, unconscious, and eventually conscious accumulation and sudden acting out of the negative countertransference that may precipitate an end to the treatment.

Once the psychopathic transference has shifted into a predominantly paranoid transference—that is, the patient's dishonest and pseudo-friendly behavior has shifted into an honest suspiciousness and distrust of the therapist—the patient may appear much more hostile and belligerent in the sessions but, by the same token, more honestly engaged in the psychotherapeutic relationship. Now the main question is the extent to which the structure of the treatment protects the patient, the therapist, and the treatment setting from the acting out of severe aggression. In other words, to what extent does the patient have a sufficiently nondestroyed, noncorrupted superego to be able to experience a minimum of guilt and concern for the therapist and the therapeutic relationship in order not to threaten the therapist or the treatment with total destruction? The task is now to examine in great detail the nature of the patient's projections, the image of the therapist that emerges throughout them as a sadistic persecutor, and, eventually, the projective processes by which the patient is attributing to the therapist that which he cannot tolerate in himself.

One patient had violent temper tantrums in connection with her suspicion that the therapist had been talking about her to third parties; she assumed that the therapist was attempting to obtain confidential information from her in order to use it against her later on. In this, as the patient gradually became aware, she was repeating the suspicious and enraged behavior of her mother, who would attempt to control the patient's communications with people outside the family and the patient's private life in general. Eventually, the patient became aware that she had been attributing to the therapist her own tendency to attempt to achieve control over other people by spying surreptitiously on them—by, for example, manipulating other people to obtain information about their parties, eavesdropping on conversations, and participating in meetings under false pretenses in order to obtain privileged information.

There are times when a patient's paranoid regression may take frankly psychotic features, with the development of delusion formation in the transference. At such points, it is important, first, to maintain the rules of strict boundaries in the therapeutic situation and to stress the kind of behavior that can and cannot be tolerated inside the hours and outside the hours; and second, to ascertain whether such delusion formation occurs only in the therapy hours or also in the patient's external life. If paranoid delusion formation develops outside the hours in a patient whose diagnosis was definitely a borderline personality organization, it is important to provide clear structure to the patient outside the hours in order to avoid dangerous aggressive and self-destructive behavior even before the nature of this behavior can be understood in the transference.

Third, once it is established that the patient's convictions are clearly delusional, the technique of "incompatible realities" may be utilized to resolve such a psychotic regression. It consists in letting the patient know that the therapist understands that the patient's conviction is unshakable, and that the therapist respects that conviction. At the same time, the therapist should add, he needs to share with the patient his own conviction, which is diametrically opposite to the patient's. The patient is thus faced with deciding whether the therapist is telling the truth or whether he is lying, and, if the therapist is lying, what that means in terms of the therapeutic relationship.

Patients who still have severe, unresolved psychopathic transferences may attribute the therapist's statement to the fact that he is lying, and then all the implications of a "dishonest" therapist treating the patient have to be explored in their transference meanings before they can be traced back to projective processes in the patient. In other words, this development reflects a regression from the paranoid to the earlier stage of predominantly psychopathic transferences. If, on the other hand, the patient believes that the therapist is telling the truth but that the therapist is totally out of reality, then the situation may be analyzed in terms of the patient and therapist occupying mutually incompatible realities—in other words, a psychotic nucleus in the transference may be circumscribed and then examined as a particular transferential problem. This approach is very effective in reducing paranoid transference regression in essentially nonpsychotic patients but is contraindicated in patients who suffer from a psychosis with paranoid features.

One patient became convinced that the therapist was presenting his comments in a sarcastic or otherwise provocative way in order to enrage her and then treat her as if she were psychotic. She, in turn, was enraged because of this sadistic, cynical, insensitive, and provocative behavior on the therapist's part. Her violent protests were condensed with her ironic mimicry of the therapist's statements, linguistic style, and accent and escalated to the point where she was thinking about making a formal complaint to the therapist's superiors. The therapist pointed out to the patient that he believed her conviction that he was treating her in such sadistic and provocative ways, but that, in his view, there was nothing in his behavior that objectively would warrant such an accusation and, regardless of what might come to light about the patient's contribution to the situation, these accusations were totally unfounded. He added that his belief required her to consider how honest he was in making such a statement and, if she thought he was honest, how he could be so blind to the nature of his own behavior as to make such a categorical statement, in total contrast with her experience of the situation. The patient, in this case, did not believe that the therapist was lying, but she could not accept that he was so blind to his own behavior that he would be unaware of something so obvious, in her view, as what she was describing. This led to the patient's acute sense of confusion and to her self-accusation that she was mistreating the good therapist. This self-accusation enabled the therapist to point out her fear of asserting a view of him that might not correspond to reality but might have an important function for her. Eventually, the patient was able to recognize in her view of the therapist the frightening experience of her "crazy" parents, who fought savagely with each other while severely intoxicated by drugs. The therapist represented a psychotic parental couple destroying their relationship and using their child (the patient) as an innocent victim of this savagery.

The working through of paranoid transferences eventually enables the patient to acknowledge the projection of his own aggressive needs and wishes and to integrate the awareness of this "persecutory" segment of his experience with the usually split-off, "idealized" segment of self-experience in which the longing and capacity for a dependent relationship, for love, gratitude, and the reciprocity of loving feelings, is sequestered. This bridging of opposite self and object representation units initiates the development of "depressive" transferences, the advanced stage of the treatment of patients with borderline personality organization.

NARCISSISTIC PERSONALITIES

We turn now from patients with significant antisocial potential to the treatment of narcissistic personalities who engage in less severe antisocial behavior and do not suffer from the syndrome of malignant narcissism. In these cases, setting up the structure that will limit antisocial behavior is usually much less of a problem. The patient's capacity for establishing a therapeutic contract is undisturbed by severe superego distortion, deceptiveness, or incapacity to accept responsibility for himself, and the main problem is the analysis of the narcissistic transferences that may occupy a major proportion of the total time of treatment.

The basic problem in the treatment of patients with predominantly narcissistic transferences is their lack of capacity to depend on the therapist, because dependency means acknowledging the importance of the therapist; such acknowledgment would generate intense conscious and unconscious envy, and, by projection, fears of the therapist's envious attacks on the patient if he does not protect himself. In addition, another major problem is the patient's massive devaluation, as an essential defense against dreaded dependency, of the importance of the therapist and the therapeutic relationship. In severe cases, the incapacity to depend may present as the patient's ongoing "self-analysis"; the therapist is treated as a "bystander," and an unrealistic therapeutic atmosphere may arise within which the therapist feels consciously (and sometimes, at first, unconsciously) excluded and frequently experiences boredom, restlessness, or sleepiness.

At other times, a primitive, frail, and unstable idealization evolves in which the patient apparently accepts the therapist's understanding or interpretations with eagerness. Over the long run, however, the patient may find these interpretations to be useless; he may also either devalue them or "extract" them as magical comments to be used for his own purposes. These patients tend to "outguess" the therapist in order to protect themselves against attacks from the therapist, against unconscious envy, and, essentially, against dependency on the therapist.

Manifestations of omnipotent control in these cases include efforts to manipulate the therapist to respond in ways expected by the patient, who also indicates that he will feel put down, humiliated, or attacked if the therapist reacts differently or proves to have any knowledge that the patient does not have himself. Alternatively, by radically devaluing the therapist's "unexpected" interpretations or statements that are contrary to his views, the patient neutralizes and, at times, ridicules the therapist. The therapist, in short, has to be as good, but neither better nor worse than the patient, and must correspond rigidly to the patient's expectations.

In addition, particularly in patients with significant superego pathology, and even in the absence of antisocial behavior, there is a severe lack of trust in the therapist's genuine interest and a suspicion that the therapist is interested only in exploiting the patient and has no authentic knowledge to contribute, only magic or quackery—in other words, "gimmicks" that the patient has to extract in order to appropriate the therapist's manipulative skills. What the patient tends to deny in the process is the therapist's distinct reality as a different human being with his own internal life. In particular, the patient profoundly envies the therapist's creativity in the therapeutic process and unconsciously needs to destroy it.

The effect of all these mechanisms may be a severe "emptying out" of the therapeutic situation, the therapist's sense that nothing is really going on, and a lack of development in the transference that obscures the fact that, to the contrary, a very active transference is developing, namely, the activation of the patient's pathological grandiose self in the transference relationship. In fact, the transitory idealizations of the therapist reflect the temporary projection onto the therapist of the patient's grandiose self-image; this idealization may be as easily withdrawn as reactivated. The patient's activation of grandiosity, omnipotent control, devaluation, and denial of dependency reflects the object relations derived from the pathological grandiose self.

When the pathological grandiose self is infiltrated with ego-syntonic aggression, the manifestations of omnipotent control, devaluation, and projective identification of all undesirable self-aspects onto the therapist become much more evident. Under these conditions, the patient may express inordinate demands, an arrogant, openly controlling behavior, and the syndrome that Bion (1967b) described as a combination of arrogance, curiosity (about the therapist's mind and life, not about the patient's own experience) and pseudo-stupidity—that is, the apparent incapacity to listen to ordinary logic and reasoning if it does not correspond to the patient's own, preset ideas. Patients given to severe narcissistic devaluation may prematurely disrupt the treatment, particularly those patients with significant antisocial features and severe superego pathology in whom the capacity for engaging in significant object relations is seriously compromised. This tendency toward early dropout needs to be differentiated from surprising, late dropouts precisely at the point when the patient has experienced the therapist as providing authentic help, in other words, when the patient has developed a negative therapeutic reaction out of unconscious envy. The therapist's awareness of this patient's potential to have such a negative therapeutic reaction may enable him to make a "preventive" interpretation of that reaction at a point when the patient seems able, perhaps for the first time, to acknowledge the therapist's help.

A careful analysis of particular aspects of the patient's grandiosity, arrogance, demandingness, and devaluation may gradually reveal the components of the pathological grandiose self, that is, the patient's condensed identification with idealized self and object representations that represent a selective takeover of those aspects of significant others that have signified for the patient strength, power, wisdom, and superiority—particularly power and superiority.

The more severe the superego pathology, of course, the more such powerful images, particularly parental images, include sadistic and corrupt features. Often patients with severe narcissistic personality who have been the victim of physical or sexual abuse or exploitation harbor a deep conscious resentment against the real or imagined perpetrators of these attacks, while unconsciously identifying with the double role of victim and perpetrator. In the transference, the activation of both victim and perpetrator status needs to be carefully explored, together with the patient's unconscious activation of all idealized aspects of past representations of self and other. Careful analysis of all these component identifications in the transference permits the gradual resolution of the pathological grandiose self and of its protective function against more primitive aggression, particularly more primitive hatred and envy. The emergence of conflicts around hatred and envy tends to veer narcissistic transferences in a paranoid direction; while, on the surface, the transference acquires much more negative aspects, in fact this trend reflects the development of a more intense and dependent object relation that lends itself to gradual working through, along the lines of the elaboration of paranoid transferences referred to earlier.

One patient tended to dismiss all the comments of the therapist that did not fit with her preset views as meaningless or stupid. At the same time, she was extremely curious about what the therapist was thinking, although she avoided talking openly about her own thoughts, fearing that open communication would lead to her exploitation and mistreatment. She also was immensely curious about the therapist's relation with his family but oscillated between resentful envy of the privileges of the therapist's family and a radical devaluation of the members of his family whom she asked about; her sense of relief was evident as she communicated to the therapist all the negative aspects of the members of his family that she had found out. Another patient, fearful that the therapist was trying to cheat him of his time in the hours, carefully checked every minute of each session in order not to be cheated, while using every pretext to prolong the hours and thus extract additional time from the therapist. This patient had the remarkable tendency to waste time in the hours, endlessly repeating the same questions and the same enraged demands for an answer, all of which tended to produce repetitively wasteful interchanges. But he would eagerly use any additional moments after the end of the session to communicate apparently important information that he had withheld during the scheduled hour. It turned out that what the therapist gave "freely" of his time and interest was worthless to the patient, and that only what the patient could incorporate by force gratified his sense of envious resentment.

One malignant expression of narcissistic resistances may be the patient's unconscious wish to defeat the treatment by destroying his own life in a gradual, undramatic, and yet highly effective way. Thus, for example, one patient successfully kept the therapist uninformed about her serious failure in her professional development—her failure to fulfill her academic responsibilities was bringing her dangerously close to being expelled from her postgraduate program—and she systematically revealed to the therapist only major crises in her professional development at a point when it was almost impossible to correct them. In the countertransference, the therapist felt called on to carry out desperate rescue efforts that would typically fail, and it took a long time before the therapist realized that the patient was successfully confusing him in order to prevent him from becoming aware of her self-destructive behavior early enough to help her correct it.

This last illustration relates to a more general dangerous development of the transference, namely, the development of "perversity" in the transference. Perversity consists in the recruitment of love at the service of aggression: the patient consciously and unconsciously tends to stimulate the therapist's dedication and commitment, to the point where the patient may frustrate that dedication and commitment and bring about failure precisely in connection with the therapist's attempts to help her. One patient stimulated the therapist to explain the nature of her problems in her relationships with men, apparently listening and applying thoughtfully the therapist's interpretations to her understanding of that particular difficulty. After several weeks of work on this problem, the patient used all that she had heard from the therapist as part of a devastating and sadistic attack on her boyfriend. In other words, she massively distorted the therapist's statements in the service of destroying the relationship with her boyfriend.

The psychodynamic psychotherapy of narcissistic resistances may be frustrating to the therapist because of the enormous time required to transform the activation of the pathological grandiose self in the transference into its component transference dispositions—the primitive object relations involved—and to gradually work them through. In its advanced stages, the treatment of these patients resembles quite closely that of other patients with borderline personality organization in whom narcissistic transferences are not dominant, and the therapist may not be aware at that point that a major breakthrough has been achieved. By the same token, the dissociation between what often seems to be the patient's active life of engagement outside the treatment situation and the monotonously narcissistic transference may prematurely discourage the therapist from gradually working through these narcissistic resistances—an essential precondition for consolidating the patient's apparent gains in the extratransferential field.

In conclusion, the most important complications in the treatment of patients with borderline personality organization arising from the combination of narcissistic, antisocial, and paranoid behaviors require that the therapist carefully assess where the patient stands along the spectrum of severity of this particular psychopathology; decide whether the patient, under the present circumstances, is at all able to undergo psychodynamic psychotherapy; set up realistic conditions and a frame for the treatment to proceed; and finally, explore and work through systematically the particular transference developments in these cases.

CHAPTER 6

The Impact of
Attachment Status

Increasingly, psychoanalytic clinicians have been applying attachment theory, which deals with the formation and disruption of affectional bonds, to understanding the therapeutic process and the therapeutic relationship, particularly with severely disturbed patients (such as borderline patients) for whom attachment issues are primary. Attachment status has been linked to the quality and nature of the therapeutic alliance (Mackie 1981), to patients' characteristic response to endings and separations (Gunderson 1990; Holmes 1996, 1997, 1998), to prevailing transference-countertransference dynamics (Dozier and Tyrrell 1998; Fonagy 1991, 1998a; Holmes 1995, 1996; Szajnberg and Crittenden 1997), and to patterns of patient-therapist discourse (Fonagy 1998b; Slade 1999). That attachment status has an impact on many aspects of the therapeutic endeavor is not surprising, since the therapist has been called the "prototypical example of an attachment figure in adulthood" (Farber, Lippert, and Nevas 1995, p. 226). John Bowlby (1977) emphasized the importance of the therapist serving as a secure base—a reliable and trustworthy person with whom the patient can explore his or her representational models of self and others so as to reappraise these models on the basis of new relational experiences. Patients inevitably bring to therapy expectations of the therapist that are consistent with their attachment histories, and indeed, the therapeutic relationship is uniquely suited to evoking and illuminating the patient's working models of attachment

93

(Kobak and Shaver 1987; Farber, Lippert, and Nevas 1995; Main 1995, 1999). By the same token, disturbed patterns of attachment can be expected to complicate psychotherapy. This chapter introduces an attachment perspective from which to view the process of psychotherapy. Although work on the relationship between attachment status and psychotherapeutic process is in its early stages, our observations suggest that attention to attachment status may help the therapist to better engage some difficult-to-treat borderline patients in transference-focused psychotherapy (TFP).

Psychoanalytically oriented clinicians are also paying increasing attention to the ways in which the therapist's feelings toward the patient, to the extent that they are non-idiosyncratic (Racker 1968), may help the therapist to understand the patient's internal working models of attachment (Fonagy 1991, 1998a, 1998b; Szajnberg and Crittenden 1997). With the more severely disturbed patient, the therapist may be able to comprehend fully the relationship developing between herself and her patient only by simultaneously responding internally to the roles induced by the patient and objectively observing these responses as a primary source of information while the patient lives out the dominant attachment pattern with the therapist.

THE BORDERLINE PSYCHOTHERAPY
RESEARCH PROJECT

As part of our longitudinal research project on the treatment of borderline patients, we have been examining the possible relationship between attachment status and treatment process and outcome for borderline patients in TFP. In this chapter, we present in detail our preliminary findings on two borderline patients that illustrate how attachment status may influence the course of treatment. We also examine how the treatment, in turn, altered their state of mind regarding attachment and their capacity for reflective thinking.

The two patients, whom we will call Adam and Beth, were in their late twenties; they had both completed at least one year of TFP with a therapist who had been judged independently to be both adherent to the manualized procedure and competent to carry it out. Both patients were diagnosed with borderline personality organization (Kernberg 1975, 1984) and borderline personality disorder according to *DSM-IV* criteria. Both had made at least one parasuicidal gesture within three months of admission to the project. Both had been hospitalized at least once and had undergone extensive, unsuccessful outpatient treatments. Further, both were considered treatment successes within the terms of the research project because they completed the year of therapy, showed diminution of symptoms, including self-injurious urges and behaviors, and demonstrated improved psychosocial functioning. To the surprise of the researchers, both were reclassified with secure-autonomous states of mind with respect to attachment in the Adult Attachment Interview (AAI) after the year of treatment (Diamond et al., 1999).

CASE EXAMPLE: ADAM

Adam was the only child in what appeared to have been a chaotic and enmeshed family. His mother was a talented musician whose career had been cut short by a degenerative chronic illness; she projected her musical aspirations onto Adam and also depended on him for emotional and physical caretaking as a result of her progressive physical deterioration and episodic depressions. Adam's brother had been killed in a car accident at the age of two in front of his parents, two years before Adam was born. His mother dressed Adam in his brother's clothes so that he would resemble him, and Adam thought she believed him to be the reincarnation of that child. Adam described his father, who was an alcoholic, as alternately cruel, seductive, and pathetic: he was physically abusive to Adam and killed the boy's hamsters on several occasions. The parents frequently separated and reunited during Adam's childhood, and both eroticized their relationship with him by engaging in a number of overt and covert sexualized interactions, including sleeping in the same bed with him.

A talented composer who was unable to work consistently and was unemployed at the time of his entry into the project, Adam said, in a retrospective account of the therapy at one year, that he had been quite wary and distrustful of his therapist in the beginning. He had let go of the "sad, tricky, lame, borderline" part of himself, however, and experienced a "gradual change of trusting her [the therapist] more." The therapist, for her part, was initially wary of Adam and doubted from the beginning whether she would have undertaken to treat him if he had not been a patient in the study. She described him as "the most creative patient I've ever had" and stated, "I've had to be on guard because it would be easy to underestimate his pathology because of that." Although she found him challenging to work with, she was captivated by certain aspects of his presentation; nevertheless, as she noted in her retrospective account of the therapy, she had had to increase her vigilance over the course of the year: "He came in a few weeks ago and said that he was writing an operetta about a well-intentioned therapist whose very interventions that were meant to try and help the patient led to his suicide. . . . Not every patient is as clever in finding ways to, you know, communicate their combination of attachment and devaluation . . . so I never know what to expect." Indeed, the clinical course for Adam during the first year of therapy was extremely variable, with periodic self-destructive gestures and actions; his self-destructiveness gradually diminished as he became involved in and committed to the therapy. He chose to continue in therapy when the research year ended.

CASE EXAMPLE: BETH

Beth depicted her family as cold and conflictual, and her embattled parents as minimally attentive and affectionate. Among her very few memories of them was that they sometimes forgot to pick her up from school. Her father was a compulsive gambler who had to file for bankruptcy several times; when not gambling, he suffered major depressive episodes. He was often absent for weeks at a time, and when present, he was sporadically violent. The family environment, according to the patient, was "just cold. . . . It was empty. . . . Everything was slate and stone, and she [the mother] just never did anything to make it warm. . . . It was just cold." As a child, Beth would retreat to an attic hideaway to comfort herself in isolation.

Beth's clinical course was relatively smooth and uneventful, despite the fact that her referral to the study was triggered by a near-lethal suicide attempt that came as a surprise to her previous therapist. When Beth entered the project, she was employed in a white-collar job that was below her capacities and was also vacillating indecisively between several relationships. Although she dutifully participated in one year of treatment and showed a diminution of symptoms and improved social functioning, her engagement with the therapist was somewhat limited and self-protective. Beth characterized the therapist as "concerned" about her and "interested" in what she had to say, but she described their relationship as "not that personal" and expressed doubts about whether the therapist really cared about her. She evoked similar feelings of disengagement in the therapist, who described their relationship as "formal and distant. . . . She would kind of close off to what I was saying and dismiss it in a devaluing way." The therapist stated that Beth "seemed to have an identification with narcissistic, cold, rejecting parents," and she felt that, after Beth chose to terminate after a year, she had treated the therapist with "the same narcissistic indifference that she felt she was the object of."

Clearly, the therapy was experienced quite differently by the two patient-therapist dyads. Attachment theory and research provide a theoretical scaffolding for understanding the differences—in the ways Adam and Beth changed during the year of TFP treatment, in the treatment course itself, in the quality of the therapeutic relationship, and in how each patient and therapist experienced each other in interviews at the end of the year. By intensively investigating the impact of patients' attachment organization on aspects of the treatment relationship and process, we hope to increase our ability to use TFP optimally. TFP offers a set of techniques and their expected progression, but it cannot be reduced to "a series of steps to be carried out sequentially irrespective of the idiosyncratic context provided by the individual patient" (Clarkin, Yeomans, and Kernberg 1999, p. 2). In this chapter, we hope to show that an essential aspect of that idiosyncratic context is an understanding of the patient's current state of mind regarding early attachment. That understanding enhances our ability to apply TFP in difficult clinical situations and is particularly important for borderline patients whose insecure attachment status may compound the clinical challenges they present.

ATTACHMENT THEORY AND RESEARCH

Attachment theory and research initially emerged from the clinical observations of the British psychoanalyst John Bowlby (1969, 1973, 1979, 1980), who was concerned about the bond that develops between child and caretaker and the consequences of this bond for the child's emerging self-concept and developing view of the social world. Bowlby (1973, 1988) theorized that early interactions with attachment figures are encoded in mental representations that he called internal working models of self and others. These working models include expectations, beliefs, emotional appraisals, and rules for processing and excluding information related to attachment. The attachment behavioral system and the internal working models that guide it continue to be significant throughout the life cycle (Bowlby 1988). Internal working models not only forecast the shape of current and future intimate social relationships but also contribute to the nature of the affects evoked and the memories accessed in those relationships (Fonagy 1998b).

Internal working models of attachment are thought to be equivalent to Kernberg's (1976, 1980) self-object-affect units, which form the basis for representations of self and others (Bowlby 1988; Diamond and Blatt 1994). Like self and object representations, internal working models of attachment are thought to reflect not an objective image of the parent but the history of the individual's *experience* of interactions with early attachment figures (Kernberg 1980, 1994b; Main et al. 1995). Bowlby hypothesized that in the course of early development the individual builds in the mind two different models: one of the self as a child in interaction with each parent, and conversely, that of each parent in interaction with the self. In his writings on psychoanalytic treatment, Bowlby (1988) stipulates that the patient may experience the therapist in vastly contradictory ways as the latter comes to represent the disparate aspects of the patient's internal working model of self and others:

> Not infrequently, a patient shifts during therapy from treating his therapist as though he was one or the other of his parents behaving towards him in the way one of his parents had treated him. For example, a patient who has been subjected to hostile threats as a child may use hostile threats to his therapist. Experiences of scornful contempt from a parent may be re-enacted as scornful contempt of the therapist, sexual advances from a parent may reappear as sexual advances to the therapist. (p. 144)

Hence, the conceptualization of internal working models in attachment theory is continuous with the object relations principles on which TFP is based, particularly the identification of the polarized representations of self and other as they emerge in the transference and the dramatic role reversals that may occur as the patient experiences both sides of the object relational pattern vis-à-vis the therapist.[1]

---

[1] Mary Main (1999) has recently commented that the term "internal working model of attachment" is somewhat misleading because it does not take into account the multiple, often contradictory working models of attachment that are found in the AAI transcripts of insecure individuals. Main (1999) and Hesse (1999) currently prefer the terms "state of mind or representational states with respect to attachment" to depict the representations of early attachment relationships that are evoked by the AAI. Henceforth, we use those terms instead of "internal working models."

Individual Differences in Attachment

Attachment status was originally classified according to the various ways in which small children were found to respond to a standardized brief separation and reunion procedure with the mother (Ainsworth et al. 1978; Ainsworth 1985). Based on Bowlby's (1977) contention that the attachment system is active "from the cradle to the grave," Mary Main and her colleagues (Main, Kaplan, and Cassidy 1985; George, Kaplan, and Main 1985) set out to assess and classify the attachment status of adults through the Adult Attachment Interview, a one-hour interview designed to assess the adult's overall representational state with respect to attachment. Main and Goldwyn's analysis of the interview led to the development of four main attachment categories, reflecting the adults' current state of mind with respect to attachment: "secure-autonomous," "dismissing," "preoccupied," and "unresolved"–of which the first three parallel the parent-child attachment patterns originally identified in children by Mary Ainsworth and her colleagues (1978) ("secure," "avoidant," and "ambivalent"), and the last parallels the disorganized-disoriented style identified in infants subjected to maltreatment or frightened or frightening behaviors by parents with histories of unresolved trauma and loss (Hesse 1999; Hesse and Main 1999; Main and Weston 1981; Main and Hesse 1990). Indeed, a number of prospective and retrospective studies have found that the adult attachment classification predicts corresponding parent-infant attachment behaviors in the Ainsworth Strange Situation (for a review, see Hesse 1999).

- *Secure-autonomous* states of mind with respect to attachment, as they appear in verbatim transcripts of the AAI, are characterized by an internally consistent and hence at least seemingly truthful portrayal of the relationships with parents in the present and in childhood; by well-organized, undefended discourse in which emotions are contained but freely expressed; and in general by the ability to discuss coherently and collaboratively both the positive and negative aspects of early attachment relationships and attachment-related experiences.
- *Dismissing* states of mind with respect to attachment are characterized by the tendency to either devalue the importance of attachment relationships or, more commonly, portray them in an idealized fashion with few corroborating concrete examples, often

accompanied by the individual's insistence that he has little memory of childhood. Inconsistencies usually emerge between vaguely positive generalizations and "leaked" evidence to the contrary.

- *Preoccupied* individuals often demonstrate an apparent freedom in talking about attachment and expressing attachment-related feelings but give incoherent and chaotic interviews marked by grammatically entangled sentences, jargon and nonsense words, childlike speech, confusion about past and present relationships, and either vagueness about parents or long passages listing their failings.

- *Unresolved* (for trauma and loss) attachment status is identified by lapses in the monitoring of reasoning or discourse when discussing experiences of loss and abuse. Although the individual's speech may be globally coherent, she either makes isolated, highly implausible statements about the causes and consequences of traumatic attachment-related events or descends into confusion and silence, followed by a shift into a discourse style indicative of a state shift such as eulogizing. Because prominent features of the secure, dismissing, or preoccupied attachment categories may surface in interviews with unresolved individuals, they are also assigned corresponding secondary classifications (for example, unresolved/ secure).

- The *"cannot classify"* attachment category signifies a more global breakdown in discourse and/or inconsistent use of discourse strategies such that the AAI shows characteristics of several different attachment classifications.

The first three categories parallel the parent-child attachment patterns originally identified in childhood (the secure, avoidant, and ambivalent) by Ainsworth and her colleagues (1978). The "unresolved for trauma and loss" category corresponds to the pattern of disorganized-disoriented attachment later described in infants who had been subjected to maltreatment or to frightened or frightening behaviors on the part of parents with histories of trauma and loss experiences about which they themselves remained (Hesse 1999; Hesse and Main, in press; Main and Weston 1981; Main and Hesse 1990).

The adult attachment categories have been found to predict parent-infant attachment behaviors in the Ainsworth Strange Situation: the "secure-autonomous" states of mind on the AAI are associated with secure attachment of the infant to the parent, "dismissing" with avoidant infant attachment, "preoccupied" with ambivalent infant attachment, and "unresolved" with disorganized infant attachment. The secure-insecure correspondence between parents' AAI classification and infants' Strange Situation response was approximately 75 percent in twenty studies in which the AAI is given after the child's birth and in prospective studies in which the parent is interviewed before the birth of the child (van IJzendoorn and Bakersmans-Kranenburg 1995; for a review, see Hesse 1999).

Attachment classifications have been found to be fairly stable over extended periods of time. Recent studies show that 64 to 80 percent of individuals assessed for attachment at one year in the Ainsworth Strange Situation and again in young adulthood on the AAI showed continuity of secure versus insecure attachment classification from infancy to young adulthood (Hamilton, in press; Hesse 1999; Waters et al., in press), although negative life events experienced before age eighteen, such as physical or sexual abuse, parental illness, death, divorce, or psychiatric disorder, were associated with significantly less stability in attachment classification (Waters et al., in press). Further research will determine the relative impact on the continuity of attachment status of other factors such as temperament, sustained relationships with family members, change-resistant internal working models, and the capacity to make use of new attachment relationships. The two examples presented here—of change in adult attachment status and in the capacity for reflective function after a year of psychotherapy—are relevant to this question.[2]

The first AAI was conducted with Adam and Beth four months into their year of participation in TFP; both were classified as having an insecure state of mind with respect to attachment, but they were insecure differently: Adam was rated "unresolved" (U) with the secondary category of "preoccupied" (E), under which he was classified according to the specific subtypes "fearfully preoccupied with traumatic events" (E3) and "angry, conflicted" (E2). Beth was rated primarily "dismissing" of attachment (D),

---

[2]The overall study, research methods, treatment technique, and assessment procedures have been described more comprehensively in previous publications (Clarkin et al. 1999; Kernberg et al. 1989; Diamond et al., in press). In this chapter, we give a brief overview of the attachment and reflective function ratings that are directly relevant to the clinical material we present.

with the specific subtype "devaluing of attachment" (DS2). It should be noted that the AAIs were coded by two separate raters, one who scored the four-month interviews and the other the one-year interviews. In addition, the AAI coders were blind to the order to administration of the AAIs and to all identifying characteristics of the patients', including diagnosis.

ADULT ATTACHMENT INTERVIEW: ADAM

Adam's dual attachment classification of "unresolved for trauma" and "preoccupied" was based on his extremely vivid, if fragmented and contradictory, AAI, in which breaks or distortions in his capacity to remember were interspersed with floods of emotionally charged memories. He did not always differentiate well between past and current experiences and gave the impression of being encumbered by his anger at attachment objects. Adam's AAI showed typical evidence of global breakdown in discourse strategies, lapses into incoherence, and loss of orientation when discussing early attachment-related traumas. Sometimes he exhibited a dramatic loss of memory related to traumatic experiences; at other times he questioned the veracity of his memories. Indicatively, he could not complete his sentences in response to the question, "Some people have memories of some kind of abuse—physical or sexual. Anything like that ever happen to you?"

> Not quite. I would say there were some close calls for sexual but not—I don't know if it would quite qualify. You know? I mean, it was all a little bit . . . I don't know. I mean, it depends on what your definition is. I mean, and they—they didn't ever like—I mean, my dad might've kicked me a couple of times or something, but I mean, they didn't like—you know—hit me consistently at all. . . . Well, just things like, um . . . like, uh, I have a memory of—you know—of my mother pulling my genitals in the bathtub like when I was . . . I don't know how old I was, I just remember—that. Because, then when I got . . . um, and you know my mom like, you know . . . was like always walking around naked . . . I swear to God . . . you know, so like they didn't—you know—do anything really, but . . .

Throughout the interview, Adam recounted such fragmented memories of physical, sexual, and psychological abuse, which continued to remain unintegrated into his adult experience and functioning. Also unintegrated was his history of loss. For example, he reported that his first experience with death was "hearing about my brother who had died . . . all the time. To the point that I thought I was my brother reincarnated. . . . And I had to start seeing like a child psychologist when I was three because I was going up to strangers on the street and saying, 'You know, my brother was killed in a car accident,' and then they'd get nervous and like laugh . . . "

Adam became disorganized when discussing attachment-related trauma and loss, and he was perceived to be generally preoccupied with early attachment relationships. In particular, he showed a great deal of current unresolved anger toward his parents:

> I do find myself swallowing so much—you know, just having to let things pass and not—stand up for myself at all about anything. Like it makes me really angry when my mother talks about going to support groups for parents of the mentally ill. It just pisses me off—I'm like, "You're the last person that should have any sort of support" . . . and even if it's true, I don't really like being categorized that way. Not by her. . . . And she does this—I mean—she's so annoying about it. I mean, she's so, you know, obviously invested in thinking of any problem I have as being purely, you know, like neurotransmitter-related. Or like, you know, biological-chemical. And she's always calling me up, you know . . . to tell me, you know, she's heard about a new drug . . . and have I thought of taking it. . . . And I'm just like, "I know you're from Indiana, and that's just the hotbed for all these kind of, you know, discoveries and breakthroughs, but, uh, believe me, it's being taken care of." . . . And I'm like, "Listen, Mom, I have a doctor!"

Also indicative of his ongoing preoccupation with early attachment figures was Adam's tendency to polarize the objects with whom he remained entangled and to seesaw between his positive and negative evaluations of them. For example, when asked to give five words to reflect his relationship with his mother, he chose *intimate, neurotic, desperate, scared,* and *confusing*. His elaboration on the word *desperate* betokens the style associated with preoccupying anger—broken and run-on sentences, undue attention to surprisingly recent or small offenses, a tendency to blame the parent for all difficulties (Main and Goldwyn 1998).

> Well, we're both kind of alternately desperate for something from each other. . . . Um, I mean, I was kind of desperate to hope . . . hoping desperately, you know, all the time that like, I don't know why but I never got used to it. . . . I

never got it in my head that she was inconsistent. . . . I always thought today would be the day everything would be like different. And she was, you know, um, very sort of—well, alternately like clingy and desperate, you know, about her relationship with me and very sort of jealous—you know, didn't like me to have friends. Um—but then, you know, that she—the next day she'd be entirely different and would want nothing to do with me.

The interview also revealed, however, Adam's nascent thoughtfulness, clarity, and reflectiveness about his relationship with his parents.

ADULT ATTACHMENT INTERVIEW: BETH

Beth had a barren and constricted manner of expressing herself in the AAI. She could recall few memories of her childhood and depicted her parents in a uniformly derogatory, detached fashion, minimized the significance of feelings linked to early attachment experiences, and generally downplayed the importance of attachment relationships throughout her interview. The words she used to describe her relationship with her mother were *cold, sometimes warm, not very motherly, calm,* and *sparse.* She could provide only the barest particulars to back up her generalizations. For instance, when asked to elaborate on *cold,* she replied by describing the physical environment of her house.

> Um, well, what really comes to mind is that she—uh, it was my—I shared a room with my sister, and she didn't . . . it was just stone. You know, there was a slate floor. My father like built our house, and everything was just slate and stone, and she never did anything to make it warm. It was like really cold.

When asked by the interviewer whether she could recall any specific memories about her mother being cold, she replied:

> No, I can't remember. It's just a feeling. I don't even really remember that much of it. It's strange, but I don't really remember my interactions with her really well. There's very little I remember.

The paucity, generality, and detachment characteristic of Beth's memories are typical when individuals are categorized as overtly dismissing or devaluing of attachment. Also typical are raw truthfulness, perceptiveness, and insight, as evidenced in other aspects of Beth's interview. When asked to describe her relationship with her father, she was more vivid and specific, saying, "It was tumultuous, scaring, loud yelling, violent, and felt guilty."

> Well, just that you never knew when he was going to erupt. Yeah, millions of memories because . . . there was always a fight—my parents were always fighting. And, um . . . you never knew what he was gonna do. I mean, sometimes he drove the car into a stone wall or he, you know, just when he was mad he just . . . or when he was going to yell at one of us, you know . . .

Although Beth showed some capacity to portray the negative or problematic aspects of her early experiences, she tended to dismiss their impact on her current functioning or development. Her tendency to distance herself from attachment-related experiences and affects is strikingly illustrated in her response to the question of how having lived with her father's episodic threats and acts of violence throughout her childhood influenced her now as an adult:

> I'm sure it must, but I don't know how really. I mean, I'm sure if, you know, if you have a great, you know, perfectly adjusted childhood it probably helps you as a result. But I don't know specifically how it affects me, but, you know, I'm sure it does.

CHANGE ON THE AAI

At one year, both patients were reclassified as "secure-autonomous" (F) on the AAI, although Adam remained on the "preoccupied" end of the secure spectrum (F5), and Beth on the "dismissing" end (F1); Adam retained the secondary classification of "unresolved for trauma." Although each achieved a secure primary status, the two patients demonstrated differential patterns of change on the AAI subscales. Both improved in ratings of overall coherence of transcript and metacognitive monitoring (the subject's ability to recognize logical errors or inconsistencies in his or her own speech); Adam's perception of his parents as rejecting, his involving anger toward them, and his denial of recall of early attachment experiences all di-

minished, and Beth showed a decrease in degree of derogation of attachment relationships and experiences overall. These findings on the AAI subscales suggest that the *trajectory* of change toward security may differ for
patients with different attachment organization.

REFLECTIVE FUNCTION RATINGS

The AAI's metacognitive monitoring subscale served as the basis for the development by Peter Fonagy and his colleagues (Fonagy et al. 1995; Fonagy
et al. 1997) of a scale to measure reflective function (RF). Whereas Main's
metacognitive monitoring scale focuses on the speaker's recognition of her
own errors in thinking or speaking and other signs of awareness of an "ap-
pearance-reality" distinction regarding personal thoughts and feelings
(Main 1991), Fonagy's scale assesses the speaker's ability to think of others
in mental-state terms, that is, to attribute intention and mind to important
others in her world. Essentially, RF is the awareness of and capacity to take
into account the mental and psychological processes underlying people's
specific behaviors; that is, to conceive of others' beliefs, feelings, attitudes,
desires, knowledge, motivations, pretenses, and so on. It is thought to result from the child's internalization of not only the image of the other but
also the ability of the other to represent the child's mental processes coherently and accurately. Fonagy (Fonagy et al. 1996) has found that the AAIs of
borderline patients are distinguishable from those of other psychiatric patients by both the rate of insecure attachment and significantly lower RF
ratings.

Adam and Beth also showed differential changes in reflective function on
the AAI. Initially, they both elicited ratings of low or questionable RF. Adam
was seen as striving to understand the internal worlds of self and other, but
concomitantly he was so overwhelmed by the power and unmanageability
of the material he related that he needed to distance himself from that very
understanding. Beth showed an overly intellectualized, somewhat abstract
sense of the mental states of attachment figures, but little of the affective resonance that might allow for fuller comprehension. After one year of treatment, Adam's reflective function shifted from low to ordinary, and he was
found to demonstrate a model of the mind of others that was easily understood and well integrated; by contrast, Beth's reflective function remained at
the low or questionable level.

THE CLINICAL PROCESS

The Impact of Attachment Organization on the Course of TFP

The attachment status of both patients was evident in every stage of the first-year TFP process: in the establishment of a treatment contract, involving the identification of problems that could interfere with the patient's safety or the therapy; in the delineation of the dominant affect themes and object relations dyads; and in the exploration of these object relations patterns and their associated affects in the here and now of the transference. Although TFP stipulates a specific sequence of treatment phases and specific guidelines for interventions in these phases, the clinical material that follows reveals that the progression from one to the next varies with the particulars of the individual patient and the unique patient-therapist dyad.

Clinical Course: Adam

The clinical course for Adam during the first year was extremely tempestuous, as would be expected given his AAI classification of "unresolved/preoccupied." It was punctuated by ongoing urges toward self-mutilation; he had to be hospitalized briefly on three occasions during the first six months. His acting out during the first year included engaging in an affair in which he played out sadomasochistic scenarios with a woman who threatened his safety as well as that of the therapist. After this stormy beginning, however, he settled into the treatment, ceased his self-destructive behavior, and became increasingly involved in and committed to the therapy, choosing to continue to participate when the research year ended.

Adam's dual attachment status of "unresolved/preoccupied" was confirmed by both his confused, fractured discourse in sessions and his chaotic outside behavior. In the initial contract-setting session, for instance, Adam tried to respond to the therapist's request that they define together the behaviors that could interfere with the treatment. He began by telling the therapist that he had contacted a former therapist three times over the weekend to tell her about his suicidality.

> ADAM: I also burned my arm with a cigarette for the first time in two years . . . and I mean, I did my best to ruin my marriage . . . I called

my wife's best friend, whom I was dating before my wife. I called, I had, I was furiously planning to call my mother ... I was thinking I was preparing to make a phone call to my mother, who's separated from my father right now, but it's back and forth, I was going to ask her if I could go home and like have an affair with her (*laughs*), like basically propositioning my mother, and it seemed like I was—like that was going to be a normal thing to do, or necessary thing to do, you know.

THERAPIST: That seemed normal or necessary?

ADAM: That it temporarily seemed reasonable.

THERAPIST: Were you sleeping or not sleeping?

ADAM: Well, I don't have any excuse ... nothing induced by drugs or anything.

THERAPIST: You see, this notion of "suicide" being the magic word is what we have to discuss ... because it's clear that it has to do with the feelings you're experiencing and from the way that you are responded to.

The therapist seems to have been momentarily derailed by the shocking, scintillating, and fragmented utterances of the patient. She went on, however, to observe that suicide for Adam represented not so much a wish "to die" as a wish to "express anger" at and to be magically reunited with others, such as his former therapist. Adam acknowledged the difficulty of relinquishing self-destructiveness, which gave expression to his simultaneous clinging to and repudiating of the significant objects in his life and was an object of attachment in its own right.

During the initial contract-setting sessions, Adam articulated his essential problem: "I have hidden from people. . . . People are dangerous." He told the therapist, for example, about feeling that he got mixed messages from his former therapist, who gave him her home number for emergency situations. But when he called her frequently in suicidal crises, she terminated his treatment and referred him to the therapy project because she found him unmanageable. Reflecting on his relationship with her, he said, "I think that, you know, in a way, you know, I feel rejected, and it makes me angry and suicidal, but being treated nicely makes me encouraged, and then it just gets confusing. . . . I mean, not that I want to be treated not nicely, but you know what I mean." Adam and the therapist then talked about emergencies and how to handle them in this treatment; in the midst of the discussion, Adam abruptly said, "Feeling miserable . . . like to die," and lapsed into an unresponsive stance. "That does sound like a chronic feeling," replied the therapist, and went on to say that Adam must have felt like he was in a state of constant emergency.

The foregoing clinical material, by necessity highly condensed, bears the imprint of the patient's "unresolved" attachment status, particularly in the lapses in his reasoning and discourse around the issue of parental abuse. Aspects of Adam's discourse are also reminiscent of the total collapse of behavioral and attentional strategies observed in the disorganized/disoriented infants in the separation and reunion task, the Ainsworth Strange Situation (Main and Hesse 1990; Main and Morgan 1996). Just as the disorganized infant freezes or plays dead upon reunion with the mother in the Strange Situation, so Adam radically halts the flow of therapeutic dialogue through his abrupt reversals and statements such as, "Feeling miserable . . . like to die," or, "Want to be dead." Indeed, Adam's alternation in sessions between a playful, witty stance and one of frozen immobility is reminiscent of the rapidly shifting and contradictory postures observed in disorganized/disoriented infants (Main and Morgan 1996).[3]

Not surprisingly, the experience of the therapist as a potentially fearful and dangerous object emerged quite quickly during an early session in which Adam talked about his parents' lack of concern for him, as demonstrated most recently when they told him that they could no longer afford to phone or visit him.

THERAPIST: Where do you imagine I'd fall on the "concerned versus not concerned" spectrum?

ADAM: Well, you're probably about where my parents are.

THERAPIST: Your parents who don't have enough money to phone you anymore?

---

[3]It is likely, given the history of loss and trauma in Adam's family, that his mother was herself "unresolved." In addition, there is evidence from the AAI that Adam showed signs of disorganized attachment as a young child (for example, being extremely preoccupied at age three or four with his brother's death). Previous research has established a strong relationship between the parent's "unresolved" attachment status and the infant's disorganization (for reviews, see Hesse 1999; and Hesse and Main 1999; Main and Hesse 1990).

ADAM: And my dad who was wondering why I didn't just jump in front of a train 'cause that would work (*laughs*). But, uh, you're not that bad.

THERAPIST: Well, but it feels that way.

Thus, an object relations pattern—cold, abusive parents and helpless, abused self—comes out early in the transference.

In the first year of treatment, Adam ricocheted between alternating representations of self as victim, victimizer, and rescuer, as caretaker of an impaired mother, and as a mentally ill person in need of care himself:

ADAM: Can I ask you a question that is so dumb, I'm afraid to ask . . . Am I mentally ill? . . . You see, my mom just gets a kick out of telling people that her son is mentally ill.

THERAPIST: Were you wondering whether I would be mom-like? . . . I think you're asking if I could allay some fear that you're having. What's the fear?

ADAM: That my mom is right. She's joined some support group [for parents of the mentally ill]. I hate the fact that it's given her something. . . . She's the one who couldn't get out of bed for weeks on end, and my father's the one who killed my hamsters, and I'm mentally ill.

Adam then produced a flood of memories about the bizarre and inappropriate behavior of his parents in his childhood.

THERAPIST: You bring up the question at the beginning of the session asking if you're mentally ill, and then you describe a lot of chaos in your family. And it sounds like at least one way to understand it is that in your mind, "Either I'm crazy or they are, but I'm not sure which is which." . . . Or alternatively, "It might be that I grew up in a crazy family, and how much am I condemned to perpetuate that."

ADAM: Well, I cannot have a family of my own. . . . I think it's the only humane thing to do. I used to want a kid desperately, but I wouldn't dare . . . 'cause otherwise I start to hope about it.

THERAPIST: It might be helpful to look at your hopes, but also at what makes it impossible.

ADAM: 'Cause I would turn into my father maybe.

THERAPIST: It sounds like you're afraid you'll turn into your father anyway.

ADAM: Right.

THERAPIST: You might be afraid that you *are* your father but you're just desperately trying to hide that from yourself. . . . It sounds like that's what your question "Am I mentally ill?" is all about—whether you're like your father.

ADAM: I'm a lot like my father.

Adam then proceeded to describe an incident the day before: he had rescued a wounded squirrel that eventually had to be put to sleep. The therapist responded: "It's interesting that right after saying you couldn't be a father, you're giving a vignette which describes a great deal of caring, but also the end result is putting some little creature out of its misery. Which is also interesting in someone who's made serious suicide attempts."

Adam quite quickly veered into talking about himself as a victimizer, telling the therapist that he tormented his wife by reminding her of his infidelities. "In fact—this is probably mean of me—I got tickets for the opera *Don Giovanni*, about a man who had lots of affairs . . . and I knew it was really in a way horrible to my wife to make her go to it with me. . . . I knew it was not really humane to have her watch it with me." The therapist wondered, "Is that part of what you meant when you said that some of you is like your father—you're saying it's like disguised aggression?"

Adam then talked about his fears that if he expressed his anger the therapist would think, "I end up angry at everybody 'cause that's what we're like—borderlines." He pointed out that he dismissed his anger by reducing himself to a diagnostic category, and that in so doing he was protecting or reassuring the therapist. Adam feared that she could not stand "the onslaught" of his anger, but the session ended with his acknowledgment that in fact she had withstood it many times. Here there is the beginning of a reappraisal or reworking of a pathological object relations pattern or internal working model, indicated by Adam's testing of his expectation that the therapist would be "mom-like" and see him as "mentally ill" or "borderline" if he expressed his painful and negative feelings, and his nascent recognition that she might be capable of accepting and containing them.

In this clinical material, we also see a rapidly alternating identification with the roles of caretaker, victim, and perpetrator. Multiple representations, each dissociated from the next, are thought to be constructed as the child alternately experiences the self in the role of rescuer, persecutor, and victim vis-à-vis parents who might themselves have experienced traumata and losses they were unable to resolve, as in the case of Adam's parents (Liotti 1995, in press; Main and Morgan 1996). In adulthood, patients whose state of mind regarding attachment is classified as "unresolved" in the AAI tend to alternate among such dissociated representations of self and other, sometimes enacting both sides of the object relations pattern. Further, in patients with a history of severe physical and sexual abuse, not only is there extreme splitting between idealized and persecutory relationships, but the relationship between victim and aggressor may become encapsulated in dissociative conditions (Clarkin et al. 1999). It is only by bringing the dissociated representations into the transference that they can be lived out, understood, and integrated.

For a long time, Adam continued to engage in destructive or self-destructive behaviors in dissociated states of which he had some awareness; he felt unable to control them, however, and tended to minimize their full significance. For example, when he got involved in acting out the sadomasochistic scenario with the abusive girlfriend, he telephoned the therapist in a panic over the situation of real danger in which he had placed himself. But he arrived at the next session light-hearted and failed even to mention the phone call until the therapist reminded him of it, whereupon he dismissed the incident as trivial.

It was not until the mutually dissociated, fragmented roles of persecutor-victim, rescuer-rescued, care giver–care receiver were experienced directly in the intersubjective context of the transference, where they could be seen as reversible, that they could gradually be integrated and ameliorated. Throughout the treatment, the therapist consistently interpreted Adam's proclivity to assume the roles of persecutor and victim and to enact them reversibly within the therapeutic arena. She was vivid and specific in identifying the inhabitants of his inner world and the ways in which they affected his behavior.

Indicatively, during the latter part of the first year, Adam accused the therapist of violating his privacy by communicating with his psychopharmacologist, even though he had known from the outset that the two would confer if he resumed medication, as he was considering doing at that juncture. The therapist affirmed that she had acted out of concern for him and observed: "You know you've described parents who mistreated you in extremely severe and inconsistent ways, and I think that is now part of you . . . and that's what's there when you are trying to destroy yourself . . . and that's what's there when you're sometimes acting with me in a way as though I have no credibility." Later in the same session, Adam said, "I am aware the times I've tried to kill myself have been extreme, and that was just an inverted version of what my father was like." The therapist then asked him how he was feeling about the treatment at that point, and Adam, who had in fact just been thinking of terminating, replied that he felt "more committed to it . . . just because of what we talked about and because I got to hold my nightmare version up to reality, and it didn't really match." Clearly, he was able to respond reflectively to the therapist's interpretation that his unresolved past experiences of trauma and abuse surfaced in the transference as situations in which he sometimes experienced himself as a victim at the hands of the therapist and at other times attacked and victimized her.

The reciprocal enactment of these object relations patterns in the transference led to their gradual clarification, amelioration, and integration, as well as to the deepening of Adam's capacity for reflective function—in other words, his capacity to comprehend the intentions and motivations of the therapist. This deepening of RF capacity enabled him ultimately to tolerate reflecting on his mother's psychological reality and on the impact on her of the death of her two-year-old son. He could subsequently talk soberly and coherently about his own fears about having children and his ability to protect them adequately.

> ADAM: I feel like I've lived through it already, and I feel like I had some past life and I know how horrible it is . . . to worry about somebody.
> THERAPIST: Or to have lost a child . . . wasn't that a big part of your early experience?

Adam began for the first time to talk about his understanding of his parents' motivations in alternately neglecting him, abusing him, and clinging to him. "I understand my parents' decision to try not to get too invested in me . . . well, they *were* invested in me, but to try not to feel caring toward me or to like me so that they wouldn't miss me." His realization that his parents' rejection and mistreatment of him stemmed at least in part from their fears and unresolved grief empowered Adam to start to differentiate his own experience from theirs. It also facilitated his acceptance of such irrational actions on his mother's part as dressing him to resemble his deceased brother. Thereafter, Adam finally began to envision and explore the possibility of having a family of his own.

Clinical Course: Beth

At the outset, Beth presented as the quintessential avoidant patient who had split off her wish for intimacy, comfort, and contact and her anger about separation. During the contract-setting phase when core problems are defined, Beth's dismissing stance surfaced in the problem she identified as primary:

> Beth: I don't like being around other people, I don't know if that . . . I haven't had many successful relationships.
>
> Therapist: I think problem number one that would come up in the therapy might be your keeping some of what you're thinking or what you're feeling to yourself. Do you agree?
>
> Beth: It's possible. I don't know. I mean I've tried to say what I'm feeling . . .
>
> Therapist: Oh, but there's some obstacle there. Because your former therapist said that you'd been having suicidal thoughts a long time before you discussed them. Is that correct?
>
> Beth: Yes.

What is most evident in the initial clinical material is the patient's strategy of diminishing, or defensively muting, her affect, particularly negative affects such as anger or sadness, in order to at once preserve and minimize her contact with attachment figures (for example, parents and therapists) whom she has experienced as rejecting and unavailable. The therapist responded to this minimization by filling in what she imagined Beth was feeling, but in a mechanical, enumerative, question-and-answer style that no reader of the transcripts of Adam's sessions would recognize as that of the same therapist:

> Therapist: But it's not so much depression, you say, it's more loss?
>
> Beth: Ah, hah.
>
> Therapist: Or feeling empty.
>
> Beth: It seems very comforting to me (the idea of suicide). That's the problem I think. . . . Even when I feel like this, I don't feel like crying.

> . . . When I'm depressed, I feel that way because I want you to know
> . . . because I don't want to be depressed anymore. . . . I just want it
> to stop.
>
> THERAPIST: So the world is a pretty bleak place?
>
> BETH: Yeah.
>
> THERAPIST: It doesn't offer much comfort.
>
> BETH: Yeah.
>
> THERAPIST: So we've got two things to look at. One has to do with the
> way that you see yourself or experience yourself . . . as being worth-
> less. And the other has to do with how you see the world, which is
> cold and very uncomforting.

These initial sessions culminated in the therapist's identification of the major affective themes and translation of them into an object relations context (the self as worthless and others as cold, rejecting, or uncomforting). That context is reminiscent of Beth's description in the AAI of the emotional climate of her family as "just cold." Indeed, in a subsequent session Beth elaborated on her conviction that expressing feelings could not possibly lead to help or affective responsiveness from caretakers. She said, "I knew it wasn't normal to try to kill yourself, but I didn't know it wasn't normal to be that depressed. . . . And it was like that in my house when I grew up, you know, it was normal to be depressed, and nobody would pay any attention to it. . . . So I guess I thought it was normal because I grew up that way."

The early therapeutic explorations revealed that Beth held back feelings not only out of her conviction that they would be discounted or ignored, as they had been in her family of origin, but also because she feared that they would be ridiculed. For example, she revealed that she had never told her fiancé about the extent of her depression. "I can remember being horribly depressed when I was with him, and I kept it a secret from him." When the therapist asked her why she had been unable to tell somebody she was planning to marry about her feelings, she expressed fear that he would laugh at her or make fun of her. One is reminded here of the observations of Main and Weston (1981) that avoidant infants are mocked or ridiculed by their mothers when they attempt to evoke attachment-related behaviors.

Variations on Beth's dominant object relations scenario (or internal working model) surfaced as the clinical material unfolded; indeed, at times the self and object images were reversed, so that Beth experienced herself as the cold, rejecting, isolative one who spurns the needy, dependent other. Her response to her boyfriend's proposal of marriage typified this reversal:

BETH: He wants to be with me more and more, and I guess I just, you know, it's kind of troublesome to me. And . . . he's gonna want to be with me all the time. . . . If he's gonna be my husband, he's gonna want to be with me a lot. And I just don't like getting tied down like that. And, you know . . . I can't handle somebody liking me that much and wanting to be near me, and right now he's like, he's sort of too much for me.

THERAPIST: Why is his wanting to be with you hard?

BETH: (*shifting her attention to the office wall*). Hey, someone changed that picture. Did you do that?

Beth deflected attention from therapeutic exploration of the issues around dependency and need stirred by her impending marriage and by the therapeutic relationship itself by focusing on the loss of the picture, like the avoidant child who concentrates on toys or objects in order to sidestep the conflicts evoked by an unresponsive mother in the Ainsworth Strange Situation (Main and Weston 1981). The therapist observed that Beth's ideal would be to marry her boyfriend but not have him around much; analogously, in the therapy her ideal would be to limit their explorations by distracting them both from the task at hand.

BETH: I don't want to be with anybody. I just don't want anybody around me.

THERAPIST: It seems like being sure somebody's there makes you uncomfortable.

BETH: I feel like I have to talk to them or something. . . . It's like everything is so buried, so deep, that I can't even get to it. I don't even know what I feel . . . and I don't even know how that happened to me. But it's like, you know, all my feelings are like they don't matter, and I don't even know what they are.

The session ended with Beth's comment on her vision of the origins of this pattern of disavowal of affect and relationships in her identification with her father's despair when he lost his job and became depressed during her childhood:

> It just did something awful to me, I don't know what it did, but it was awful. I felt so bad for him. I felt for him what he felt, which was totally—he couldn't function anymore after that. . . . He never really worked again after that. So, you know, I pretty much had to fend for myself after that, you know. . . . And that just made me very upset. . . . And I just never really got over it, you know. . . . He wouldn't deal with it . . . very hopeless.

This statement identified another major self-object scenario involving a depressed, hopeless, dysfunctional other in interaction with a self-sufficient, coping, but overburdened self that might underlie her defensive foreclosure of feelings and the importance of relationships. In the second half of the therapy year, the object relations scenarios of the neglected, scorned child and the rejecting, ridiculing parent, and the ineffective, despairing other and the overburdened, competent self, were enacted reciprocally in the transference in a more direct and sustained way. By this point, Beth was more forthcoming about her depression and about her anger at her parents. In the context of talking about the suicide attempt that had led her former therapist to terminate treatment with her, Beth expressed her contempt and derogation of need for relationships. "I don't know, all I know is the last thing I wanted was my parents to be around, or my sister, I didn't want anybody. . . . (*snickering*) No. I don't want anybody around, it makes me sick, I don't want, ugh." The therapist commented that her suicide attempt might have represented her wanting more from her former therapist. Beth insisted that there was nothing that anyone could ever offer her to alleviate her feelings of depression, besides an extra phone call, which is what her therapists had given her in the past.

THERAPIST: I don't think that's what you really wanted in your heart.
BETH: I don't know what I could possibly want in my heart.
THERAPIST: Maybe more than an extra phone call or so.
BETH: What could someone give me besides an extra phone call? There's nothing else to give me.
THERAPIST: Well, what do you give your parents when they need it?
BETH: I'd do anything for them.

THERAPIST: That may be part of what gets you depressed and angry.

BETH: But I don't want anybody to do that for me. To me, it's embarrassing that people know I'm depressed. I don't want—I would never tell anybody . . . it's embarrassing . . .

THERAPIST: So how do I understand your telling me today (*that she was depressed*), since you said you wouldn't tell anyone?

BETH: Because you're my doctor. . . . I mean, I want you to somehow say, "Oh, you're depressed," and, "I want to help you," or, "I want to feel bad for you," or something . . .

THERAPIST: I want to do something.

The activation of Beth's self representation as neglected and unworthy of care alternates in this material with her expressions of scorn and disgust toward the therapist and others who want to offer help or comfort. Throughout the second half of the year, Beth's intractable dismissiveness increasingly evoked compensatory hypervigilance on the part of the therapist.

According to Beatrice Beebe and Frank Lachmann (1998), mothers of infants who fail to sustain gaze or respond robustly to their vocalization and are later classified as avoidant attempt to facilitate interactions by means of intrusive behaviors. Beebe and Lachmann hypothesize that the therapist of the avoidant patient sometimes adopts a compensatorily overzealous stance not unlike that of the mother trying to engage the avoidant toddler. The intense tracking attendant on such a stance heightens the risk of dyadic misregulation because it lessens the focus on internal states of self and other. The avoidant patient may consequently experience the therapist as "intrusive, shadowing or suffocating" (Beebe and Lachmann 1998, p. 502), even while also welcoming the therapist's persistence in making emotional contact (as with Beth's evident ambivalence).

Throughout Beth's treatment, the pattern of the neglected, ridiculed child and the rejecting parent was addressed over and over again. But in part because significant dynamics of relating were reenacted rather than explored in the therapeutic dyad—in particular the evasion of contact in order to ward off a hypervigilant caretaker—Beth decided to terminate even though she had benefited from the treatment in many respects. Her decision to terminate was in part a result of the reenactment on the procedural level for both patient and therapist of the scenario associated with dismissing attachment.

THE PATIENT-THERAPIST RELATIONSHIP

The clinical process vignettes suggest that the same therapist can engage in qualitatively different ways depending on the nature of the patient's state of mind with respect to attachment. Excerpts are presented here from the Patient-Therapist Relationship Interview (PTRI). This interview, which was adapted from the AAI, asks both parties to reflect on the relationship with and representation of the other at one year.

PTRI: ADAM

In keeping with his AAI rating of "unresolved for trauma" and "fearfully preoccupied," Adam asserted that he was not "forthcoming" with his therapist, whom he thought was uninterested in helping him and would forget about him between sessions. He noted that initially he endeavored to shield himself from the intimacy of the relationship and from feeling known by her because "I thought I was somehow defending myself against something and at the same time was wasting time, of course. . . . But, uh, it was worth it to me at that point."

Adam's description of how over the course of treatment his therapist came to serve as a secure base for him is reminiscent of Bowlby's (1988) conceptualization of the relationship between patient and therapist:

> I guess I feel a little more secure in general just because she has been so reliable as a steadying influence. . . . I kind of feel like I survive the unreliable things in day-to-day life better because there's something that's sort of steady. And just having one thing (or I guess I should say another thing, because my wife is also pretty reliable) that is kind of safe helps with all the things that aren't safe. The way a home would ideally feel when you're a kid.

Asked to supply five words that reflected his current relationship with his therapist, Adam chose *reliable, dignified, important, mildly frustrating,* and *confusing.* He was able to support his descriptions with semantic memories. As an example of his being important to the therapist, he described how he called her upon receiving a threatening phone call and felt reassured by her prompt response and soothed by her reminder that they could explore his reactions at greater length in their next session. Reflecting on what separations from the therapist were like for him, he said that while they were "stressful" and at times "seemingly endless," they became progressively easier for him to manage. When asked what he does when he's upset, he replied that he tends to talk about it a lot, but he no longer tries to kill himself—which he states he "got out of his system." He summed up the changes in their relationship by saying that he had gradually come to trust her more. At the end of the first year, Adam chose to remain in treatment and negotiated a fee for continuing; by that time, he had a job and could contribute to the cost.

The therapist was initially wary of working with Adam and reported that she had felt alternately uncomfortable, frightened, angry, exasperated, or threatened. At times she became flooded and confused, her disorganized response echoing Adam's own response to his seductive, overstimulating, and abusive parents. She acknowledged that she attempted to contain these feelings by redoubling her attention to setting up a treatment contract and renegotiating it when necessary. However, despite his history of near-lethal suicide attempts and the tempestuous initial phase of treatment, the therapist experienced Adam as engaging and even captivating, as evidenced from the five words she chose to describe him at one year: *committed, stable, creative, interesting,* and *somewhat enjoyable*.

The examples she gave in support of these descriptors indicated that her experience of Adam was rich and multitextured, if often confusing and contradictory. When asked what separations from him were like, she recalled that whereas he had made his former therapists miserable before and after vacations, his behavior was now less chaotic. She in turn was not overly anxious about his safety. When she thought about Adam on occasion when away, it was less with trepidation than with pleasure or curiosity about his communications. She summed up the experience:

> I think more than any other patient he's made me aware of how creative a borderline patient can be, and how you have to be careful not to underestimate the pathology because of that. . . . My way of looking at it, and I've said this to him, is that he seems to want to have the sessions as though it's a Jane Austen novel, with all the sophisticated charm and humor, but under the surface there's a Steven King novel lurking, and you can't forget about that.

In the context of a treatment that provides a high degree of structure and consistency and preserves the therapy as an arena for the exploration of the underlying conflicts that fuel acting out, the patient with an "unresolved/preoccupied" attachment status may be quite engaging, if challenging, even while requiring the therapist's vigilance.

PTRI: BETH

Just as Beth had described in the AAI growing up in a cold and stark environment, so did she experience the treatment relationship as distant and uninvolved. She described her therapist as helpful and competent, but she was unsure whether the therapist was really emotionally engaged with her or whether she was just doing her job as a therapist. "I think of her like a doctor . . . like, I come in, I do my work with her, and I leave. . . . I don't know if I really think about her a lot when I'm not here. Occasionally I think maybe if I was having a hard time I thought maybe I wanted to talk to her or something . . . but nothing stands out in my mind." As is characteristic of individuals classified as dismissing, she described her therapist in generally positive terms but had difficulty backing up her descriptions with specific examples. When asked to choose five words that reflected their relationship, she said *very professional, understanding, controlled, concerned about me,* and *not that personal.* The few episodic illustrations were paltry and unconvincing. On the therapist's concern for her, for example, she said: "I think she was always concerned—like she always seemed interested . . . you know, in what I was talking about."

Beth minimized the significance of separations from the therapist and reported not feeling anything when informed about an upcoming vacation. Her first response was, "I didn't really feel any . . . you know, no problem." Then she added, "Maybe there was once or twice when I maybe got depressed when she was away and I said to myself that I couldn't wait till she came back, . . . But I didn't really miss her greatly when she left." When asked how the therapist responded when she was upset, she added, "She'd . . . give me an idea of why I was feeling the way I was feeling . . . um, I didn't get that upset this year." As to her choice to terminate therapy at one year, Beth reported that she felt "a little sad," but only for "a week or two" afterward. But then she added, "It's gonna be weird not to see her twice a week every week. . . . I miss her a little bit."

We can surmise from the PTRI that one contributing factor in Beth's decision to terminate was a desire to protect herself from the difficult feelings stirred up by the therapy. She reported that the therapy definitely helped her and made her "realize more about myself . . . why I do things and why I feel the way I feel sometimes and, you know, where it comes from." However, this focus on affect made her feel exposed, particularly when the therapeutic explorations challenged her tendency to distance herself from the threat of attachment-related information or from the affective experience of relationships, including the therapeutic one. For instance:

> Sometimes it made me mad almost because things I wanted to be a secret sort of, if I was angry about something. I didn't want her or anybody to know I was angry. . . . Consciously, I didn't know I didn't want anybody to know, if you know what I mean. But she'd say or start digging into things and find out why I was angry, and then I'd realize something really made me mad, but I didn't want to be mad. With my parents, for example, I didn't want to be angry at them.

The heightened anxiety and insecurity that Beth's statement communicated has been associated with a shift from "dismissing" to "secure" attachment organization (Hazan and Shaver 1994).

The therapist was somewhat constricted and inhibited in discussing Beth. Consistent with the findings (Dozier 1990; Slade 1999) that the dismissive patient often evokes countertransference feelings of rejection and exclusion from the patient's life, the therapist stated:

> I don't think she ever wanted me to see everything going on inside of her, so she would be well behaved and withholding at the same time. . . . It was hard for me to try and keep in mind . . . or figure out how to get to the deeper levels, because she would go on about manifest-level issues, problems with her job . . . and I was always looking for an angle to get in deeper. Which, of course, I could find—we did make some progress with that. But on the whole, I'd say that the relationship was formal, distant.

In addition to having felt dismissed by the patient, the therapist recognized that Beth probably experienced her as dismissing, or at other times as intrusive. When asked how she thought Beth felt about her, the therapist replied, "I think she probably thinks I'm a nice person and a good therapist, but [someone] who was a little overzealous and was trying to make more of her than was really there."

When asked to choose five words to describe her relationship with Beth, the therapist picked *distant, rigid, formal, cold,* and *superficial.* Citing an example of the distantness, the therapist remembered that Beth came in one morning and announced, "I'm getting married this afternoon." Although the therapist had known that Beth was engaged, she reflected that "usually a person's a little more . . . just a little more is made of their marriage." She felt that more than anything this incident "encapsulated the way she was so . . . out of touch with affect." The therapist noted that Beth would treat separations as though they were "nothing"; when she announced that she was going away, Beth would say, "That's fine, okay, no problem."

The therapist said that she rarely thought about Beth outside of the treatment situation, and that she had no fantasies about her. Reflecting on their relationship, she asserted, "Nothing could ever get to her or touch her or evoke a reaction from her." Acknowledging that she felt rejected and disappointed by Beth's decision to leave treatment after one year, she understood it as Beth's way of "turning the tables" on others by whom she had felt "chronically dismissed."

> She seemed to have an identification with narcissistic, cold, rejecting parents who left her feeling very tenuous about her claim on, you know, just being alive. . . . She always seemed to feel like an afterthought and resented not being more of a priority in the lives of people. . . . She seemed to be extremely wary of any connection to anybody because it didn't register to her that it could be real, and so she walled herself off in an isolated, protected state and simultaneously, without much awareness, treated people with the very narcissistic indifference that she felt she was the object of.

DISCUSSION AND CONCLUSIONS

Two patients with the same diagnosis and level of personality organization but with very different internal working models of attachment engaged the therapist's subjectivity in vastly different ways, leading to a different treatment course and outcome. Although clearly the attachment status of each patient influenced the quality of the relationship with the therapist, Beth's stance was experienced as the more formidable. The therapist's response to her dismissiveness, pursuing her elusive affects, served to increase her dismissiveness. It is important to note that Beth made some substantial gains during the treatment year. That she made no suicide attempts or gestures, was not rehospitalized, and made a commitment to one relationship and got married could all be seen as resulting from the diminution of identity diffusion and improvement in object relations expected during the first year of TFP (Clarkin et al. 1999). Despite these gains and symptom stabilization, however, Beth's treatment process led to an impasse: the therapist was unable to work reciprocally and flexibly with her projections. Indeed, Beth externalized in the therapist intolerable aspects of her internal world and early attachment history, as evidenced by the unilateral and somewhat polarized nature of the five words the therapist chose to describe her relationship with Beth at one year: *distant, rigid, formal, cold, superficial.* Thus, the therapist's experience of the patient was configured through projective identification to represent an aspect of the patient's internal world—notably, the dismissing state of mind with regard to attachment.

By contrast, Adam's "unresolved/preoccupied" dynamic found a fuller, richer, and more nuanced resonance. The therapist readily tolerated even his most heinous projections and near-violent enactments, along with the welter of pleasurable and frightening feelings he evoked, and was able to contain and use them to therapeutic advantage. Like Bion's (1967) model of the container and the contained, the therapist's work with Adam metabolized and detoxified his projected affects, impulses, and internal states and presented them to him in more tolerable form to be reexperienced and reinternalized. Thus, the therapeutic process, with its inevitable projections and introjections between patient and therapist, was reversible and at times playful, as indicated in the five words that the therapist chose to describe her relationship with Adam at one year: *committed, stable, creative, interesting,* and *somewhat enjoyable.*

Reflective function is so fine-tuned a measure of the capacity to comprehend and explore the mental contents and processes of self and other that it provides a particularly sensitive gauge of not only the therapist's and patient's capacity to assess their mutual experience but also of the therapeutic outcome. That Adam's reflective function increased significantly in the AAI while Beth's did not change is consonant with the fact that both Adam and the therapist showed a greater degree of understanding, flexibility, and reflectiveness in their retrospective accounts of the treatment on the PTRI than was the case with Beth. These findings strengthen our sense that different relationships may bring into ascendance different representational states with respect to attachment for both the patient and therapist. We might hypothesize that the improvement in Adam's reflective function at one year derived in part from his internalization of the therapist's vivid and coherent internalized representation of him, whereas the lack of improvement in Beth's reflective function resulted in part from the therapist's difficulty in reflecting flexibly and vividly about her mental states and processes.

It is clear that attachment classifications can serve the therapist as a guide to understanding the implicit relational knowing or procedures (Lyons-Ruth, 1999; Stern et al. 1998) that form the bedrock of current interaction patterns or forms of narrative discourse. Such a conceptualization adds another dimension to the task of the psychoanalytically oriented clinician—to monitor the aspects of therapeutic interactions that may contribute to intensifying or diminishing the patient's insecure attachment strategies.

Attachment classification goes beyond psychopathological diagnosis to highlight individual differences in response to treatment interventions and prepare the clinician for them. Although attachment categories may amplify diagnostic understanding, the clinician in practice must remain attuned to the subtleties of transference that may manifest in secure, dismissing, preoccupied, or unresolved configurations in keeping with both the patient's history and the current interactions in the therapeutic arena (Lichtenberg, 1999).

However, given the substantial evidence offered by attachment researchers of the continuity through the life cycle and across generations of internal working models of attachment, it is not surprising that aspects of the treatment experience and relationship are initially assimilated to their configuration (Main et al. 1985; Hesse 1999). Attachment classification can function as a guide for the therapist to the nature of the problems that will first emerge in psychotherapy, the early transference-countertransference dynamics, and the probable response to endings and separations, permitting technique to be used in an appropriately nuanced manner.

It is important to note that not all aspects of these patients' presentation or of the therapeutic transactions can be reduced to or understood in terms of attachment concepts. Much more research and clinical observation needs to be done on how attachment status converges with different forms of pathology, different levels of organization, and different diagnoses (for a review of recent work in this area, see Hesse 1999). For example, it is clear that severe identity diffusion or lack of consolidation of an internal sense of self (Diamond et al., 1999; Foelsch and Kernberg 1998) helped to configure and perhaps intensify Beth's dismissing dynamics.

Nevertheless, attachment concepts, whatever their limitations, are expanding the boundaries of psychoanalytic understanding and treatment of severely disturbed patients. The AAI, although relatively new to use with clinical populations, has been shown to be a reliable and valid instrument for assessing constructs related to borderline personality organization, as well as for empirically investigating aspects of psychoanalytic process and outcome (Fonagy et al. 1995, 1996; Hesse 1999; van IJzendoorn and Baker-mans-Kranenburg 1996).

Although attachment research provides evidence that new experiences and relationships later in life can alter a person's internal working models or state of mind with respect to attachment, these models of attachment have been found in numerous studies to be quite stable over time and resistant to change. We were surprised that Adam and Beth were judged by independent blind raters to have shifted their attachment status from insecure to secure after only one year of TFP, given the severity of their pathology and our experience that it generally takes years of treatment before such patients are able to make substantial long-term change. We were expecting subtle changes on the subscales rather than gross changes in overall classification. We may surmise that the shift to secure status indicated improvement in the organization and coherence of the patients' verbal discourse and in their capacity to use such discourse to cope with and express impulses and affects that they had been expressing through self-destructive acting out.[4] Additional findings on the ways in which changes in attachment classification were paralleled by a decrease in levels of symptomatology, particularly in self-injurious impulses and actions, provides support for these formulations (Diamond et al. 1999). Although deeper dynamic changes, including the consolidation of changes in internal working models of attachment, have probably yet to occur, the increased coherence and reduction in symptoms in these patients after one year speak to the power of TFP to effect structural and behavioral change.

Of course, it is also important to consider how the therapist's own state of mind regarding attachment (which we did not evaluate) and idiosyncratic

---

[4]According to Mary Main (personal communication, 1999), at four months, when the AAI was first given, these patients demonstrated some capacity for the type of fresh, open, lively, perspicacious recounting of early attachment experiences that is associated with the secure/autonomous representational states. This renders their reclassification as secure at one year less remarkable.

countertransference influence the treatment course. The former is a particularly important area for further investigation in the light of Mary Dozier and Christine Tyrrell's (1998) recent finding that although secure states of mind in therapists are more likely to produce good clinical outcomes, the therapist's location on the secure spectrum (from "dismissing" to "preoccupied") affects treatment success: therapists at the more "dismissing" end of the secure spectrum showed better clinical outcomes with "preoccupied" patients, and therapists at the more "preoccupied" end showed better clinical outcomes with "dismissing" patients.

However, even given these limitations, our findings suggest that attachment theory and research will broaden and sharpen the theoretical lens through which we view aspects of the therapeutic process and the patient-therapist relationship.

CHAPTER 7

Schizoid States and Paranoid Regressions

Schizoid states are personality configurations in which splitting is the primary defense and defensive operations centered on the patient's fantasy world replace those involving intense interpersonal involvement. Affects in particular are often split off from cognition. The borderline personality organization is divided into personalities that rely on interpersonally based defenses, like projective identification and omnipotent control, and personalities that are characterized more by introversion, preoccupying themselves with fantasy and employing defenses primarily in that realm. The former category comprises such personality disorders as the borderline personality disorder proper, the histrionic personality disorder, and the hypomanic personality; included in the latter category are the schizoid, schizotypal, and paranoid personality disorders. Schizoid states pose special problems in the conduct of psychodynamic psychotherapy because of its reliance on a transference focus. Moreover, as treatment progresses and schizoid patients begin to engage the interpersonal world, they may suffer paranoid regressions that must be managed in the treatment. This chapter examines the special considerations involved in the treatment of schizoid states and paranoid reactions.

SCHIZOID STATES

Bleuler (1908) and Kretschmer (1925) offered the first comprehensive descriptions of the schizoid state, emphasizing the detached facade, attention

129

to inner reality, and lively but contradictory inner world. Behaviorally these individuals are aloof, cool, and suspicious. They desire solitariness and often exhibit vague life pursuits. At times they can be highly involved in social movements, although usually of an idiosyncratic nature. Usually they remain detached and on the fringes of society and may describe themselves as drifting or floating through life. Their aloofness and confusion are often accompanied by a moral arbitrariness, and these individuals sometimes exhibit odd or criminal behavior.

A major contradiction exists between this external facade and the individual's subjective state, which is one of hypersensitivity and vivid experience. These individuals may exhibit odd or magical thinking and frequently display a rigid cognitive style. Thought processes are greatly valued, and there is a preoccupation with primitive fantasies, often of a grandiose or paranoid nature.

From a dynamic standpoint, these contradictions between internal and external states, as well as between emotional sensitivity and detachment, are best explained in terms of defensive management of primitive anxieties. Melanie Klein (1946) was one of the first to describe the intrapsychic dynamics of schizoid individuals, detailing the mechanisms of splitting and projective identification that allow for the disavowal of emotional states. These processes are employed, in Klein's view, to manage infantile persecutory anxieties that derive from inborn aggressive drive energy. Although primitive defenses characterize borderline pathology in general, the schizoid state is earmarked by two specific features: the dramatic splitting off of affect, giving rise to what Fairbairn (1940) described as the "deemotionalization" of object relations, and the substantial elaboration of fantasy. Unlike Klein, Otto Kernberg (1995, in press) suggests that schizoid personalities do not make extensive use of interpersonally enacted defenses, such as projective identification.

Fairbairn also described an attitude of omnipotence in both the fantasies and the interpersonal relations of these individuals. He hypothesized that early life frustrations resulted in fixation on and overvaluation of part-object representations, with a preference for taking over giving in the individual's emotional life. Schizoid individuals report being exhausted after social contacts and have immense difficulty sharing emotional responsibility in relationships. At the extreme, the "as-if" personality of Deutsch (1942), or D. W. Winnicott's (1960) "false self," describes the detached exterior put forth by these individuals.

In diagnosing the schizoid state, the therapist should keep in mind the underlying theme of profoundly contradictory emotional states. Akhtar (1992) provides an excellent description of how schizoid phenomena manifest in the domains of self-concept, interpersonal relations, social adaptations, cognitive style, and intrapsychic structure. Schizoid individuals see themselves as stoic, self-sufficient, compliant, inferior, and as outsiders. Interpersonally they are aloof and fearful of intimacy and have few close friends. They prefer solitary activities, occupationally as well as recreationally. Schizoid individuals appear to be asexual and rarely become romantically involved. Cognitively they may be absentminded, preoccupied with fantasy, and prone to stilted speech. In contrast to these overt manifestations, strikingly different covert characteristics of the schizoid individual may become apparent during the course of intensive treatment. These include preoccupation with hidden grandiose or vengeful fantasies, great interpersonal sensitivity, hidden desires for closeness, vague or fluctuating personal goals, the capacity for creative and sustained work in some areas, and secret voyeuristic and perverse interests.

For a more comprehensive review of schizoid mechanisms, the reader is referred to the works of the authors mentioned earlier. In brief, it is hypothesized that all individuals exhibit schizoid phenomena at some level of their personality. In those individuals for whom primitive aggression is unmanageable, schizoid mechanisms may predominate and manifest at all levels of functioning. These individuals feel that their aggression can destroy those they love, and they are prone to developing a compulsion to hate and be hated as a defense. Primitive defenses of splitting and projection are used to destroy intrapsychic object relations in an effort to disperse intense affect states. Although these individuals appear externally distant and aloof, they have an immensely active internal life. Thought processes are greatly valued, and the dispersal of object relations is accompanied by a preoccupation with primitive fantasies, often of a grandiose and/or paranoid nature. These fantasies are manifestations of the primitive splitting mechanisms and represent a massive failure of integration.

In the clinical setting, schizoid phenomena manifest in a variety of ways. In early treatment, the therapist will recognize these states when the patient reveals fantasies highlighting contradictory attitudes toward close emotional ties. Themes of love-as-destructiveness accompanied by defensive wishes to both hate and be hated are central and, as noted already, are at the core of much of borderline pathology. Although identity diffusion is present, countertransferences do not resemble those seen in severe states of identify diffusion, where a sense of confusion predominates. The countertransference to schizoid patients instead often involves concordant feelings of distance and coldness in the therapist. Deeper examination of transference and countertransference phenomena reveal a massive dispersal of all object relationships and a splitting off of linking affects, leaving only occasional, fleeting emotional states.

TECHNICAL INTERVENTIONS

Because schizoid states are relatively fixed and chronic, there is usually no need for acute intervention. The standard TFP techniques of clarification and confrontation can be used to elicit the primitive fantasies described earlier. This uncovering process may take an extended period of time given how extensively splitting is used by these patients. When evident, these splitting mechanisms should be interpreted; affect-laden, primitive fantasies should then emerge. In borderline patients without narcissistic or antisocial traits, an extended period of clarification of these fantasies will ensue. With ongoing confrontation and interpretation, the patient will gradually experience some integration of disparate object relations. The patient may then experience great relief and become more able to describe the severe anxiety states that accompanied the schizoid state. Because of this, the therapist should be careful not to interpret worsening anxiety as a sign of clinical deterioration.

One of the problems encountered in psychodynamic treatment of schizoid patients is difficulty in utilizing the transference. Although schizoid patients readily incorporate the therapist into their fantasy life, they avoid affective involvement with him in the hour. When a part-self-object dyad is activated in the transference, the linking affect is split off. As a result, the emotional reality of the interaction is lost. This makes it more difficult for the therapist to identify the central transference paradigm activated in the moment and to take advantage of the transference to demonstrate to the patient his internalized part-self and part-object representations. With the affect missing, the therapist may have more difficulty in identifying the particular representations activated in the transference.

One helpful technique is for the therapist to be watchful for indicators of split-off affects in the session. To maximize the effectiveness of transference work, the therapist should remain vigilant for linking affects of the transference that have been split off and appear elsewhere in the session. Such affects may be found in the patient's behaviors in the session and, especially, in his fantasies. Thus, one patient quietly sobbed while coolly describing his relationship to the therapist in a manner in which there appeared to be no basis for sadness. Another patient, who had great difficulty experiencing anger toward the therapist, reported the fantasy of striking the therapist with his car as he was driving to the session. The fantasy was reported with little affect; an interesting curiosity, as though it had no real meaning in terms of his feelings toward the therapist.

The identification of such disconnected affects in work with schizoid patients is central. Once the therapist has spotted a split-off affect, he should use it as a guide to help identify the active transference state. Before directly addressing the transference with the patient, the therapist should begin by calling the patient's attention to the split-off affect and encouraging her to wonder about its disconnection from the content of the session. The therapist may then explain the meaning of the affect as it serves to link the part-self and part-object representations he has identified in the transference, and the defensive function served by splitting it off. In work with schizoid patients, identifying split-off affects and reconnecting them with the part-self and part-object representations in the transference is a central therapeutic tactic.

Only by repeatedly linking the affect back to the transference can the therapist demonstrate to the patient that connectedness to the therapist will not lead to destruction. Gradually the transference will take on a more real quality, and the patient will begin to make better use of transference interpretations.

In working through chronic schizoid states, the therapist may uncover primitive narcissistic or antisocial traits. As the patient's capacity to experience affect increases, she may begin to withhold information or even actively deceive the therapist. Such deception arising during the psychotherapeutic work with a schizoid patient should be regarded as a sign of antisocial personality in someone who does not otherwise have antisocial features. It is also common to uncover primitive narcissistic fantasies at this stage, especially the fantasies of omnipotent control originally described by Fairbairn (1943).

PARANOID REGRESSIONS

Analysis of schizoid states often leads to acute paranoid regressions. This is because the patient's aggression becomes more threatening to him as he allows himself to get closer to other individuals. Projective mechanisms are then needed to export the persecutory aspects of the self into others. Since schizoid patients, like narcissistic patients, are particularly focused on themselves, they may also defend against their aggression by erecting a grandiose self—perfect, pure, and well behaved. Thus, schizoid states may shift into narcissistic ones. There is often an initial oscillation between narcissistic and paranoid features; interpretive work may initially intensify the paranoia.

Paranoid regressions are not unusual in the treatment of borderline patients and appear in the absence of schizoid states as well. When projective identification is intense, patients may project persecutory self representations onto the other person, provoke the other to be sadistic, and then, in the process of identifying with the other, reintroject a now intensified original sadistic object. This cycle of projection and introjection of intensified persecutory part-objects, truly a "vicious cycle," can blur the boundary between self and other and open the way to transient psychotic distortions and paranoid regressions.

When paranoid processes emerge in the treatment of the borderline patient, the therapist must make a careful differential diagnosis of the paranoid process. Paranoid traits, as distinguished from acute paranoid regressions, are often encountered at some point in the treatment of borderline patients. This is the individual who appears to have been "dropped behind enemy lines." He is vague and unrevealing and meets inquiries with counterattacks and accusations. Some borderline personality organization patients present with paranoid features and may meet *DSM-IV* criteria for paranoid personality disorder. Other patients present with predominantly narcissistic and/or psychopathic features, and paranoid traits emerge in the course of psychotherapy. In other instances, which we discuss soon in more detail, acute paranoid regressions are encountered that may threaten the continuity of treatment. They are often unexpected and intense and are characterized by sudden persecutory rage and accusations.

In paranoid regressions, the activated part-object relationship is one of torturer and victim. This object relationship can manifest at any level of psychosexual development. Anal-sadistic elements are seen when the patient describes the therapist as withholding and greedy. At other times, the patient may feel that the therapist is overwhelming and devouring, exhibiting oral features. Oedipal-level reactions are seen when the patient accuses the therapist of competing with her in an effort to harm or defeat. The more disturbed the patient, the more primitive the activated relationship. Condensation of images and collapse of levels of psychosexual development can be seen, for example, when a patient accuses the therapist of harboring wishes to rape her as a means of destroying her efforts to achieve autonomy and self-control. Also, rapid role oscillation is seen as representations of persecutors and victims switch. The therapist may witness the patient first feeling like the helpless victim of attack and then becoming a vicious attacker of the therapist.

Paranoid fantasies around primitive aggression can also involve the superego or infiltrate the dynamics of love relations. In the former, sadomasochistic fantasies emerge (see the discussion of sadomasochism in chapter 4); in the latter, the patient may express erotomanic transferences. In these situations, the patient is convinced that the therapist is in love with her and may inform the therapist that any statement otherwise is a lie. Paying attention to a history of previous paranoid experiences, including their duration, intensity, and eliciting circumstances, will help the therapist to assess paranoid states in the transference. Also, any early and sudden transference reactions should be closely explored with the aim of making a differential diagnosis. Later in treatment, specific transference and countertransference reactions will give the therapist clues as to which type of paranoid reaction he is encountering in the patient.

DIFFERENTIAL DIAGNOSIS

The most important judgment to be made when the therapist initially encounters paranoid ideation is whether it is indicative of a psychotic process. Three psychotic states are the most common: a previously undiagnosed Axis I psychotic illness, such as schizophrenia or bipolar disorder; a brief psychotic reaction; or an acute transference psychosis. The crucial distinguishing factor is the patient's capacity to reality-test. A psychosis is diagnosed when the patient reports hallucinations or delusions and is consistently unable to identify the "as-if" quality of the symptoms, or when the patient is unable to empathize with the therapist's perception of ordinary social reality. During one structural diagnostic interview in which the interviewer revealed little of himself and elicited the patient's transference reaction, the patient reported that she felt the interviewer was planning to rape her during the interview. To assess her capacity to empathize with his sense of ordinary social reality, the interviewer asked the patient whether she felt this was a likely possibility given that the interview was being conducted during midday in a centrally located interview room in a busy hospital setting and was being videorecorded. The patient ignored all of these reality elements and replied that she remained as frightened as ever that the possibility of rape was real. She could not empathize with the interviewer's sense of all the reality factors that served to safeguard her in this situation. This patient, although initially diagnosed as borderline, turned out to have a bipolar psychosis.

In assessing a paranoid reaction, the therapist should also consider whether there are acute *precipitating events* and whether the psychotic symptoms are confined solely to the *transference*. If there is no acute precipitating event, and the symptoms generalize beyond the transference to the patient's whole life situation, there is a strong likelihood that an underlying chronic psychotic illness has been uncovered. (See chapter 3 for illustrations of psychotic illnesses misdiagnosed as borderline.) If there is a precipitating event and the patient's psychosis generalizes, then a diagnosis of reactive psychosis should be considered. For example, after a man who had worked as a city building inspector was laid off from his job, he developed the conviction that his coworkers had intensely disliked him for some time and had told the false story to the FBI that he took bribes on the job. For weeks after his dismissal, he remained convinced that he was under police and FBI surveillance. When the precipitating event is a treatment-related occurrence such as the surfacing of an intensely warded-off affect, memory, or realization or a perceived abandonment by the therapist, it is more likely that the psychotic state is *regression in the treatment*. The psychosis may be entirely focused on the therapist, as in the case of the patient who became convinced that her therapist cleared his throat in a derisive manner whenever she had a good feeling in the session in order to undermine her chances for happiness in life. This is indicative of a *transference psychosis*.

In brief psychotic reactions, precipitating events can be identified, one of which includes intense transference reactions. These are states of acute and severe emotional turmoil with psychotic symptoms that are not necessarily confined to the transference. In contrast, an acute transference psychosis in a patient with a borderline personality organization is confined to the transference and usually consists of specific hallucinations or delusions. Auditory hallucinations are common. For example, a patient in the midst of a paranoid transference psychosis may hear the therapist derisively calling his name during the session or at other times in the day. Other hallucinations can be encountered as well. The patient may see the therapist's face or claim to smell disgusting odors coming from the therapist during sessions. Delusions of persecution are also very common in transference psychoses.

A final distinguishing factor is the intensity of the psychotic reaction. In a transference psychosis, the symptoms evolve gradually and require much exploration before they surface, as opposed to brief psychotic reactions or schizophrenic episodes, in which the symptoms emerge suddenly and with great intensity.

TECHNICAL APPROACHES

Because of the intensity of paranoid regressions, especially psychotic reactions, the therapist must consider safety issues. The risk of both acute and chronic dangerousness in the patient should be assessed by noting: any history of violence; the degree of present impulse control; whether there is concurrent substance abuse; the degree to which superego functioning is intact and the capacity for a moral stance; and physical factors that influence the assessment of dangerousness. (For example, a tall muscular young man is more of a risk than an elderly frail woman.) If there is a risk of real threat, the therapist should not hesitate to suggest interrupting the treatment for a consultation or hospitalization, with the possibility of resuming when the therapist feels safe to continue the work.

If the situation is less clear and the therapist is uncertain whether there is a risk, she should immediately raise the issue with the patient. The therapist may say, "Before we go on, it looks like you're tempted to harm me. Can you assure me you have these impulses under control?" If assured that the patient is in control of any violent impulses, analysis of the reaction should ensue. Otherwise, limits should be set as necessary. If there is any possibility of risk, patients should not be seen in off hours or in isolated treatment areas. It should always be clear to both the therapist and the patient that treatment will stop if necessary at any time.

It is crucial that the therapist always be clear and direct when analyzing paranoid reactions. The more timid the therapist, the more likely it is that the patient will sense a great fear of his aggression and be unable to manage and explore the fantasies. When a relaxed, direct therapist gives the message that the primitive aggression can be managed, the patient's anxiety diminishes.

The following example illustrates how an acute, psychotic paranoid regression in the transference is managed.

CASE EXAMPLE

Ms. F. was a twenty-seven-year-old woman with a borderline personality organization and a narcissistic personality functioning on an overt borderline level. Her main difficulties were chronic suicidal behavior, severe incapacity to maintain any work situation in spite of having obtained a master's degree in the field of music, and chaotic relations with men that evolved rapidly into severely sadomasochistic interactions and eventually ruptured, resulting in the practical absence of any gratifying, stable sexual or love relations. She evinced a chaotic lifestyle, reflected in her drifting from one subordinate job to another, weathering severe affect storms, and chronically fighting with her entire family, from whom she had become practically isolated; at one point, she almost became a "street person."

The sessions with Ms. F. had been marked by intense affect storms. She rejected practically everything the therapist said and distorted his statements so that they would become an immediate attack on her; she complained endlessly about his coldness, indifference, invasiveness, and cruelty; and she described the warm, friendly, understanding, and spiritually uplifting quality of her previous therapies. It needs to be mentioned that most of these therapeutic encounters were of brief duration, except the one with a psychotherapist who practically adopted Ms. F. and blurred the boundaries between therapy and personal friendship. The treatment with the present therapist was now in its second year, the longest she had remained in a treatment situation. In the context of this treatment, she had been able to take up and maintain a job more commensurate with her knowledge and experience for the first time in her life. The suicidal attempts had stopped, her impulsive and chaotic relations with men had decreased, and the relationship with her family had become less stormy, but it is no exaggeration to say that "all hell would break loose" in most of Ms. F.'s sessions with the therapist.

To summarize the outstanding dynamics of her case, Ms. F.'s mother was a chronically alcohol-dependent person who had committed suicide during the patient's childhood. Ms. F.'s father was an effective school administrator who had tried to "discipline" his youngest daughter, who, in contrast to her older siblings, became a major source of concern for him because of her severe behavioral disturbances from early adolescence on. He tried to interfere with her chaotic sexual life, and she experienced him as both intrusive and jealous of her relations with other men.

In the transference, from early on, Ms. F. alternated between times of violent and complaining behavior, exhibiting a haughty grandiosity and pseudo-stupidity that seemed to reflect closely Bion's description of the syndrome of arrogance (Bion 1968), and other times when her behavior was subdued, complaining, yet subtly seductive and she presented herself in the session in minimally acceptable clothing and engaged in clearly exhibitionist behavior. Early interpretations had focused on her fear that only a caring father could protect her from the callous indifference in her relationship with her mother, but that such a concerned father would invariably become sexually seductive and exploit her. Ms. F. reported no history of sexual abuse, and it was not difficult to interpret her fear that any concern of the therapist for her would seem like sexual exploitiveness as a projection onto him of her own wish to seduce her father—the only alternative to the catastrophic unavailability of her mother. In simple terms, she perceived the therapist either as intrusive, invasive, and potentially sexually seductive or as cold, indifferent, and lethargic.

In recent months, this behavior had shifted into ever more intense rage attacks in which she accused the therapist violently of not listening, of distorting what she said, and of imprisoning her in the treatment. She seemed totally impervious to all his interpretations. She attempted to throw objects at him and managed to damage minor objects in his office, and on a few occasions, the therapist had to warn her forcefully that any further damage to any object in the room or physical attack on him would mean the immediate end of the session. She learned exactly what her limits were and often would stand in front of him shaking her hands and yelling at the therapist.

The present session started with just such a development of intense rage and yelling. The therapist pointed out to Ms. F. that she had left the last session talking with him calmly about a problem at work, and he indicated that his help to her in sorting out her emotional reaction to a colleague had helped her to decide how to handle the situation. He wondered whether she now had to create a "scene," and was attempting to provoke him into a rage, because of her own experience of hatred and violence as expressions of profound guilt over the implications of having moments of a good relationship with him. In response to this comment, Ms. F. got much worse, accusing the therapist even more of total ignorance, distortion, and lack of memory of what had happened in the last session and of focusing only on her relationship with him rather than on the terrible problem she had to face at work every day.

The therapist then commented that she was feeling much worse after he had pointed out that she maintained a fighting situation because of the intolerance of the memory of good moments of her work with him. He wondered whether now she felt that he was trying to make her feel guilty over how she was treating him after the good relation that had evolved in the last session. Ms. F. interrupted him several times and, in apparently repeating what he said, distorted his words completely. At that point, the therapist, in a strong voice, told her that in his view she was talking sheer nonsense and that he assumed that, although she was attacking him as if he were hostile and indifferent, that this was completely false, and that, in his view, point by point, in what she had just said she had distorted everything that he had said. The therapist insisted that, while he understood that she was totally honest in attributing to him an aggressive and indifferent behavior, in this perception she was attributing to him something that had absolutely nothing to do with where he really stood and represented an attribution to him of her own behavior that was not motivated by any real behavior from him, as far as he could see.

The therapist, in pointing out the "incompatible realities" of her perceptions and his own at this point, was probably also acting out, in part, his frustration with Ms. F.'s ongoing attack, but mainly he was focusing on the complete incompatibility of the views they each had of his behavior. In a later reflection on this moment of the session, he said that, though he had partially enacted the hateful, persecutory object she had unconsciously projected onto him, he had reacted mostly as the victim of a sadistic, overwhelming, invasive, hateful object and, in pointing to the "incompatible realities" of their perceptions, attempted to make Ms. F. aware that she was enacting the hateful, attacking object of which he now had become a victim.

In fact, following this intervention by the therapist, Ms. F., to the therapist's surprise, responded thoughtfully, and in a totally natural voice, that he could not tolerate her affect storms: Wasn't the treatment geared to permit her to express herself freely in the hour? After recovering from his surprise, the therapist said: "I am impressed by the fact that you can talk to me in a normal way only after I talk to you as loudly and perhaps as harshly as you talked to me before. I wonder whether this is a confirmation that you cannot tolerate it if I talk to you in a thoughtful, calm way, as if talking to an adult, rational woman, or maybe that only when I yell at you can you really believe that I care." The patient had been taking his relatively calm delivery of his interpretations, he suggested, as "indifference or phoniness."

Now Ms. F. remained silent; after a few minutes, she started to cry. She said that he did not know how much she was suffering. The therapist wondered whether perhaps the only way in which she felt able to let him know how much she was suffering was in attempting to provoke him with hateful behavior, so that he could experience the sense of impotence and paralysis that she sometimes experienced herself at work. Shortly after this exchange, the hour ended.

This case example illustrates, in part, how a therapist can utilize the technique of sharing with a patient his perception of the "incompatible realities" between the patient's experience and the therapist's experience, although it also illustrates a partial acting out of the countertransference induced by the projective identification of a primitive, hate-dominated, persecutory object.

Most probably, the relationship between a sadistic object and its victim— possibly a very primitive layer of experience reflecting the deeply disassociated hatred of an unavailable mother or the relationship with a "drunken" mother who could be aroused only by violence—had been enacted in the session. What did not occur, however, was the reversal of this relationship, which might have been expected as the consequence of the partial acting out of the therapist's countertransference. To the contrary, Ms. F. was able, for the first time in the session, to register the therapist's communication to her—an illustration of the effectiveness of the method of communicating "incompatible realities" as part of the interpretive approach to severe paranoid distortions in the transference.

CHAPTER 8

Depression and Suicidality

In carrying out psychodynamic treatment of borderline patients, the therapist almost invariably encounters depressive states. This is because the borderline patient struggles with the brutality of internalized persecutors that devalue, induce primitive guilt, and destroy. The use of primitive defenses prevents the moderation of affect, leaving the patient vulnerable to severe depression. These defenses also make use of the interpersonal impact of depression to influence important others in the patient's life. Specific personality disorders within the borderline personality organization may be particularly predisposed to depression, and borderline patients may be at increased risk for inherited affective syndromes as well. Suicidality is a frequent complication of the borderline personality disorder. On the other hand, depression may reflect important progress in treatment as the patient's representations of self and others become more integrated.

Addressing the complications introduced by depression and suicidality requires a careful diagnosis of the sources of these states, an assessment of risk, and the selection of interventions appropriate to the type of depressive or suicidal state. Depending on the nature of the depressive state, intensive interpretive work, particularly with a transference focus, attention to the countertransference, medication, limit setting, intervention in the patient's life, and hospitalization may each play a role.

SIGNS AND SYMPTOMS OF
DEPRESSION IN THE BORDERLINE PATIENT

Borderline patients may display any of the symptoms associated with major depression, dysthymia, atypical depression, masked depression, or normal depressed mood. Some such symptoms of depression are more characteristic of borderline personality disorder than others. These include feelings of emptiness and chronic loneliness, fears of abandonment, preoccupation with interpersonal losses and separations, self-destructive behaviors, self-condemnation, angry neediness, and involvement in demanding, hostile, dependent relationships (Gunderson and Elliott 1985; Rogers, Widiger, and Krupp 1995). On the basis of their study of twenty-one borderline patients, Rogers, Widiger, and Krupp (1995) also report that hopelessness is more characteristic of depression in borderline patients than other depressed, personality-disordered patients. Conscious guilt, remorse, and withdrawal from others, on the other hand, are more characteristic of unipolar depression.

The primitive defenses of the borderline patient may influence the ways in which depression manifests in the session. Because of the activity of splitting defenses, the conscious experience of depression may be kept separate from depressive thoughts or motoric expressions of depression. It is not unusual for the therapist to observe in the borderline patient an apparent disconnection between cognitive reports of depression, behavioral signs of depression, and vegetative symptoms. Sometimes tears come to the eyes of the borderline patient during the session, but he has no awareness of depressing thoughts or affect, only of some feeling of perplexity. The powerful borderline defense of projective identification can cause the patient's depression to become manifest first in the therapist rather than in the patient. The therapist may, for example, feel a sense of hopelessness or of giving up, or intense sadness. The patient disavows his intense hopelessness and depression by evoking those feelings in the therapist and maintaining the belief that it is the therapist, not the patient, who has given up.

At times the depressed affect is accompanied by a sufficient number of symptoms to meet criteria for diagnosing an Axis I affective disorder. In such cases, the depression may represent a true mood disorder. The rote application of *DSM-IV* mood disorder criteria, however, can be misleading. It is also possible that the patient's description of symptoms may be stereotyped, exaggerated, or overly simplistic, giving the impression of an Axis I syndrome when closer inspection reveals a more characterological depression.

Histrionic character features, for example, may lead a patient to describe a depression as unrelenting for weeks at a time, so that it apparently meets the *DSM-IV* criteria of depression "most of the day nearly every day for two weeks or more," when in fact the depression waxes and wanes and is interrupted for extended periods by social attention or romantic interest. Similarly, although the narcissistic patient may describe persistent depressive feelings of failure and worthlessness, close inspection may reveal that the depression dissolves each time he experiences success or praise.

Paying attention to the symptom's stability, duration, and the interpersonal context in which it occurs may be necessary to differentiate characteristic Axis I symptoms from transient, situational, or exaggerated symptoms. It is particularly helpful to examine depressive symptoms in interpersonal contexts. Characterological depressions tend to fluctuate, varying with opportunities for social contact or the influence of external stimuli, and may disappear when the patient is distracted. Patients with major depression sometimes feel worse when others try to cheer them up. Patients with dysthymic disorder are typically unable to shake the heavy feeling.

Sources of Depression

Comorbid Affective Disorders.   Borderline patients may indeed have a concurrent Axis I affective disorder that emerges or recurs during psychotherapy. In an outpatient clinic sample, Hagop Akiskal (1981) reported that almost two-thirds of borderline patients had a concurrent affective disorder at the time of index evaluation. Prevalence rates for affective disorder in borderline patients ranging from 14 percent to 83 percent have been reported (Gunderson and Elliott 1985; Zanarini et al. 1998). Although inpatient and outpatient studies report comparable overall rates of affective disorder among BPD patients, major depression is more prevalent among inpatients (Pope et al. 1983), and dysthymia, cyclothymia, and bipolar II disorder among outpatients (Akiskal 1981). It is important to note, however, that patients meeting the descriptive *DSM-IV* criteria for dysthymia may represent two subgroups: those with a mild chronic variant of Axis I depression and those with characterological depressions (see the discussion of depressive personality predispositions later in the chapter). Nevertheless, in spite of the high prevalence of depressive symptoms in borderline patients, John Gunderson and Katherine Phillips conclude in their review (1991) that BPD is not simply a variant of depression. The prevalence of depression in BPD may arise in part from biological features common to both disorders and in part from a reaction to the interpersonal consequences of borderline pathology (Koenigsberg et al. 1999). The depressive symptoms in borderline patients can arise from many sources other than the affective syndromes of *DSM-IV, Axis* I.

Borderline Mechanisms.   In the borderline patient, depressive symptoms often result from the activation of particular internalized part-object relations. During the early phase of treatment, before integrated ego and superego structures have formed, depression frequently reflects an attack by a bad part-object representation on a part-self representation. Aspects of significant figures in the patient's life, experienced as sadistic because of their actual behavior or because the patient has imbued them with her own aggression through projective mechanisms, may become internalized persecutors. Such persecutory part-objects may lead the patient to berate herself, to hurt herself, or ultimately to attempt suicide.

When the patient has experienced a good object as frustrating because it does not provide sought-after gratification, she faces the dilemma of hating a needed object. This may lead to a defensive idealization of the frustrating object and a devaluation of the self (Jacobson 1971), stimulating feelings of inferiority or worthlessness. Alternatively, the patient's intense need to be in control may be projected or activated in others through projective identification, leading her to experience herself as totally controlled by others and therefore to feel helpless. Feelings of aloneness may result when the patient's aggression is turned against the representations of needed objects in her internalized world, destroying them as potential sources of comfort.

One patient would periodically complain of intense feelings of loneliness, guilt, and depression over some weekends during a particular phase of her treatment. After a while, it became apparent that these feelings emerged in the treatment once the patient had begun openly to criticize the therapist, whom she had purely idealized up until then. In fact, it was specifically during the weekends that followed her attacks on the therapist that the patient felt the most intense loneliness. There were no changes in the availability of her friends and relatives over this time. As this pattern began to surface in the treatment, the therapist was able to suggest to the patient that her weekend depressions came from the feeling that her critical comments had destroyed the therapist in her mind, hence she felt more intensely alone. This interpretation resonated with the patient; she produced confirmatory associations and the weekend loneliness soon subsided.

In some instances, the patient's attacks on good internalized objects, in turn, may bring about severe intrapsychic punishment from sadistic introjects acting as a primitive superego. As a result, the patient may have diffuse feelings of badness and worthlessness.

Some borderline defense mechanisms rely on activating feeling states and behavioral responses in others. Omnipotent control is predicated on inducing a particular behavior in another person in the service of assuaging some unconscious anxiety. Projective identification reinforces the patient's projection by actually inducing another person to play the role that the patient requires to be projected onto him. One of the most powerful interpersonal imperatives is the depressive cry, an urgent request for relief from suffering. It induces strong feelings in those who are in a close relationship with the depressed person. As such, it can be the mechanism through which the borderline defenses of omnipotent control and projective identification are put into play. A patient's complaint of unremitting misery may induce guilt in the therapist that he is not doing enough, or it may make the therapist feel powerless or inadequate. In this way, the patient's own feelings of powerlessness, worthlessness, or guilt are disowned and placed within the therapist through the mechanism of projective identification.

Personality Predispositions.   Within the borderline personality organization, certain personality constellations predispose to depressive symptoms. Those with narcissistic personalities are prone to depression whenever they are forced to confront a discrepancy between the pathological grandiose self and the real self. Routine setbacks and disappointments call attention to how they have fallen short of their grandiose aspirations and provoke depression. The process of growing older, with its narrowing of possibilities for unlimited future successes and its accompanying decline in physical abilities and attractiveness, often induces depressive states. Feelings of worthlessness and powerlessness may surface. The patient, becoming aware of the shallow nature of his relationships, may feel intense loneliness and despair. In addition, narcissistic personalities have impoverished superegos that are dominated by persecutory superego precursors. Attacks by these severe introjects intensify the depression. Narcissistic patients may also become suicidal in an effort to compensate for their feelings of powerlessness: seizing on suicide is an expression of ultimate power over life and death.

Histrionic (infantile) personalities and patients with borderline personality disorder proper are also particularly susceptible to acute or chronic depression. These patients are characterized by lability of affect, overdramatization, self-centered and clinging object relationships, and promiscuous sexual behavior, motivated primarily by dependent and exhibitionistic needs. They may have suffered early maternal deprivation or significant separations or illnesses in the first years of life, leading to an intensification of oral-level conflicts. As a result, these patients are prone to feelings of low self-esteem, depression, and helplessness (Zetzel 1968). Interpersonal losses or separations stimulate intense feelings of worthlessness and depression in these particularly rejection-sensitive patients.

Depression is also commonly seen in sadomasochistic personalities. These patients form close and dependent relationships in which their behavior oscillates between self-abasement and sadistic attack on the partner. This is the consequence of sadistic internalized representations that attack the self, attack others, or are projected onto the other, leading to the experience of being badly treated or abused. Under the onslaught of their internalized attacker, sadomasochistic personalities feel demeaned, debased, and inferior.

Although depressive-masochistic personalities do not have a borderline structure and so would fall outside the scope of this chapter, familiarity with this character type is important to distinguish it from the borderline character types that present with depression. Depressive-masochistic personalities do not make use of primitive defenses, and their object representations are whole and three-dimensional. Their depressions derive from an excessively strict but well-integrated superego. They tend to be excessively hard on themselves and are serious, dependable, and overly conscientious. They are influenced by powerful unconscious guilt and have difficulty permitting themselves pleasure. Sometimes they must suffer in advance as a price for pleasure. Overdependent on others for support, they seek out displays of love and sympathy to which they can respond with gratitude and reciprocated love. Depressive-masochistic patients have difficulty expressing aggression and often become increasingly depressed rather than overtly angry.

Environmental Factors.   Borderline patients live turbulent lives. Their maladaptations lead, not infrequently, to realistic disappointments or failures in the settings of work and love. Relationships may be lost, career progress disrupted, and economic stability compromised, leading to hardships in living. Such setbacks, disappointments, and hardships may be expected to give rise to depressive feelings in their own right. In addition, the defenses used by narcissistic, histrionic, *DSM-IV* borderline, and sadomasochistic personalities rely heavily on the use of others for mood regulation. This makes these patients especially vulnerable to disruptions of important relationships.

Furthermore, borderline patients often use psychoactive substances to eradicate unpleasant feeling states or to obtain intense gratification. Many of these substances—alcohol, cannabis, benzodiazepines, barbituates, opiates—may produce depression, which may also develop after the use of stimulants (cocaine, amphetamine, diet pills) during the immediate post-intoxication period.

Depression Accompanying Improvement.   As the use of such primitive defenses as splitting diminishes over the course of treatment, the patient forms integrated and less caricatured representations of others. People become more complex and three-dimensional, and the patient is better able to empathize with others. At this point, she comes to recognize that the very therapist who has been the target of such intense rage does in fact possess good qualities, like patience and understanding. The patient now is able to feel empathy for the pain that she may have caused the therapist during periods of angry attack, and she begins to experience genuine regret, remorse, and guilt, leading to depression. But this is a depression that signals the beginnings of identity integration, that is, the development of integrated self and object representations; it can be distinguished from the more pathological depressions by its self-reflective quality and its appearance in the context of a deepening of object relations. The more pathological depressions, on the other hand, have an interpersonally rejecting quality. With the emergence of the depression of the advanced phase of treatment, the patient becomes able to utilize the therapist's understanding to feel better, something that was not possible in the earlier phase of treatment.

With the development of integrated representations of self and other, the psychic structures of ego and superego form; a more neurotic organization develops, and with it the possibility of associated depressive states. Conflict between superego and ego may develop, and guilt appears in a less primitively punitive form. Ambivalent feelings may be experienced toward persons in the patient's life. Their loss may lead to identification with their undesirable qualities and self-condemnation for this in place of conscious aggression toward them—in other words, melancholic loss (Freud 1917). A final source of depressed affect as recovery progresses is the anticipated termination of treatment; the patient begins to mourn the loss of the therapist and the treatment.

DIAGNOSING DEPRESSION
IN THE COURSE OF TREATMENT

When depressive symptoms are present in a session, the therapist's task is to diagnose the primary sources of the depression and to decide on the approach to take. Because so many sources may contribute to depression in the borderline patient in treatment, it is helpful to take a systematic assessment approach and to consider five vantage points in diagnosing the depressive state: biological, phenomenological, characterological, transferential, and environmental.

In exploring the biological domain, the therapist should assess the extent to which classical neurovegetative symptoms are present. These include weight loss, decreased appetite, amenhorea, decreased sexual interest, insomnia (particularly early morning awakening), constipation, feeling cold, psychomotor retardation, and diurnal mood variation. The presence of a strong family history for affective disorder or alcoholism is also suggestive of a biological component to the depression. Finally, careful consideration should be given to whether the patient may be using depressogenic psychoactive substances.

The therapist should next look closely at the phenomenology of the symptoms. Have reported symptoms been present continuously over a period of weeks at a time, or do they come and go over periods of hours? Are the depressive symptoms highly reactive to the social environment, or are they relatively fixed? Can the onset and offset of the symptoms be related to events in the patient's daily life? For example, some borderline patients experience an intensification of depression specifically in relation to their psychotherapy sessions. Is there merely a subjective sense of fatigue or decreased concentration, or do these symptoms actually compromise the patient's capacity to work? In evaluating the patient's reported symptoms, the therapist should take into account the patient's expressive style: Is the patient histrionic or prone to exaggeration? Is there secondary gain associated with appearing depressed?

To determine the characterological contribution to the depression the therapist should diagnose the specific personality within the borderline organization. Those particularly vulnerable to depression include the narcissistic, histrionic, and sadomasochistic personality disorders; the depressive-masochistic personality, which may emerge late in treatment, is also associated with depression among patients who achieve a neurotic organization. The task is made easier for the therapist who is working intensively with the patient, because he has greater opportunities to observe characteristic defense patterns and recurrent transference configurations, as well as to monitor his own countertransference reactions. We briefly summarize here the clinical features that distinguish these personality types. (For a more detailed discussion of their differential diagnoses, see Kernberg 1984, 1992; and Akhtar 1992).

Patients with narcissistic personalities may be identified by the predominant use of idealization and devaluation as defenses. They experience themselves as unique, special, and superior, deserving of special privilege and tribute. They may be manifestly grandiose, or they may hide grandiosity behind pseudo-humility. Their relationships tend to be shallow, and they show little capacity for empathy. When faced with disappointment or failure, intense feelings of worthlessness emerge. Narcissistic patients struggle with their aspirations for inordinate success and are prone to intense feelings of envy for others who succeed. In the countertransference, the psychotherapist feels irrelevant or ignored by the patient, as though invisible. Boredom may arise in the sessions, or the therapist may struggle with secret feelings of envy for the patient.

The histrionic personality, like the narcissistic, presents as self-centered but is capable of a greater degree of emotional involvement with others. The relationships of the histrionic patient are characterized by dependency and may be quite clinging. Histrionic patients are emotionally labile, dramatize their feelings, and are often manipulative of others. They appear childlike. They may be promiscuous, seeking to gratify primitive dependency and exhibitionistic needs through overt sexual behavior. Unlike the healthier patient with a hysterical neurosis, the patient with a histrionic personality displays a more caricatured sexuality. Although the countertransference of the therapist treating a hysterical personality may be marked by feelings of genuine sexual excitement, the pseudo-seductiveness of the histrionic patient has a socially inappropriate quality to it that is less apt to induce sexual feelings in the therapist. The therapist may witness the patient going through the motions of a seduction, yet not feel seduced.

Patients with a sadomasochistic personality alternately attack others and debase themselves. They aggressively complain of mistreatment by others and experience themselves as victims. Projection of their own aggressiveness gives them a paranoid worldview. They are "injustice collectors" who employ apparent victimization as a weapon while keeping alive their own feeling state of having been humiliated. Sadomasochistic patients attack themselves as relentlessly as they do others. Since these patients make use of their own suffering to attack others, they are prone to negative therapeutic reactions; getting worse as treatment progresses becomes a way of hurting the therapist.

Depression emerging during the course of psychotherapy may reflect the affective tone of the current transference. The depression may be a reaction to a perceived slight or failure by the therapist. A separation from the therapist, however brief, may stimulate depressive states. Holidays, vacations, weekends, or even individual missed sessions may contribute. Depressive symptoms may be more likely at such times when the transference has strong dependent or counterdependent features, or when the patient experiences herself in a victim-victimizer relationship with the therapist. Since suffering and complaints of unremitting depression have powerful interpersonal effects, they may function in the service of defenses that rely on controlling the other (namely, omnipotent control and projective identification). Thus, depressive symptoms may be invoked to keep the therapist close, to induce him to gratify the patient, to make him feel impotent, or to attack him. By understanding the state of the transference at the moment, the therapist can better assess the extent to which depressive symptoms may be intensified or dramatized to influence the therapeutic relationship—until, in the later phases of treatment, the patient may experience genuine guilt for having attacked or overly burdened the therapist.

Finally, in assessing the depression the therapist should remain cognizant of the patient's life situation. Depressions in healthier patients may be fairly obvious reactions to losses, role transitions, ongoing interpersonal disputes, or a paucity of social relationships, but the splitting characteristic of borderline patients may keep aspects of the patient's current social reality out of the session and the therapist's awareness. The patient may fill the hour with emotion-laden material about one sector of her experience but make no reference to serious negative changes in her life situation that may in fact be responsible for her depressive feelings. The therapist should maintain an awareness of the patient's external life circumstances, particularly in the spheres of work, family, social relations, and leisure. If he finds himself in the dark in any of these areas, he should consider whether the patient is using splitting defenses to keep material about her life out of the session. Interventions to clarify the external reality or to interpret splitting may be called for to bring information into the session so the therapist can take into account the effects of life circumstances on the patient's feeling state.

Clinical depressions arise from varying admixtures of characterological, interpersonal, situational, and direct biological influences. To assess the relative balance among these components, the therapist should attend to the phenomenology of the symptoms, the character structure of the patient, and the patient's social environment. The greater the extent of depressive characterological predispositions and environmental reactivity, the more likely it is that there is a significant characterological component. The greater the prominence of neurovegetative symptoms and the greater the intensity and rigidity of the depression, the more likely it is that there is a significant Axis 1 component. Many patients have an acute depression superimposed on a chronic depression, that is, *double depression.* In such cases, the chronic component may reflect either a characterologically based depression or a depressively biased neuroregulatory system, and the acute component may indicate either a major depressive episode or a reaction to events in the transference or the patient's social environment.

In sum, depressions that emerge during the psychotherapy of borderline patients may stem from a variety of sources and are difficult to assess. Combining a careful phenomenological approach to symptoms with attention to biological signs, characterological predispositions, the current state of the transference, and current life circumstances is essential in understanding such depressions.

TACTICAL APPROACHES
TO DEPRESSION

When a biological component is suspected, the therapist should consider a trial of antidepressant medication. Dysthymic disorders as well as major depressions are responsive to a variety of antidepressants. The introduction of medication during intensive psychotherapy with borderline patients is a complex undertaking, for the recommendation of medication is apt to be viewed through the distorting prism of the current transference, and the therapist's wish to introduce medication itself may be determined by countertransferential factors. The medication may acquire particular symbolic meanings. Sensitivity to side effects and compliance with the regimen are likely to be affected by the dynamic processes heightened in the course of the psychotherapy. Evaluating the effects of medication is difficult because of the difficulty in factoring out the effects of transference, opportunities to use the medication as a vehicle for primitive defenses, and mood fluctuations secondary to the affective instability characteristic of borderline patients. Introducing medication can also provide a cleavage line for additional splitting. The integration of medication into psychotherapy is discussed further in chapter 12.

When dysthymia has been diagnosed in the absence of major depression, a reasonable case can be made for either introducing or withholding antidepressant treatment. Patients meeting *DSM-IV* criteria for dysthymia may fall into one or both of two subgroups: those with predominantly characterological depression and those with imbalances in their neurotransmitter systems. The latter may be expected to respond to antidepressant medication. Since the effectiveness of antidepressants can usually be assessed in a period of three to six weeks, a trial of medication is one tactical option for dysthymic borderline patients; the medication can be discontinued after six weeks or so if the results are negligible. Initiating psychotherapy without medication is an alternative option for this population, particularly when characterological features are prominent; by avoiding the complications of a combined treatment, the therapist can observe whether the depression responds to transference-focused interventions.

When external circumstances or life events contribute to depressive states, they should be acknowledged. Expression of sympathy for major losses may be entirely appropriate. The patient's feelings and reactions should be clarified, and care should be taken not to pathologize reactions consistent with the circumstances. Thus, even though a woman's primitive pattern of interaction may have driven her husband to insist on filing for divorce, her grief at the loss may be an entirely normal reaction. It should be recognized as such, independent of separate efforts that might be made later to understand how the patient came to drive her husband away. In situations where splitting has been used to keep external reality out of the treatment, this should be explored, confronted, and interpreted.

Case Example

Once the role of external events and neurochemical influences has been taken into account, the therapist addresses the depressive symptoms by examining the dyads of part-self and part-object representations that have become activated, since depression may be an affect linking a particular self and object representation. The dyads are examined by clarifying the transference and by exploring interpersonal vignettes described by the patient—as illustrated in the following transcript of a session early in the third year of the psychotherapy of a depressed woman in her thirties with a borderline personality disorder and a sadomasochistic character type. Specifically, the therapist used the techniques of clarification, confrontation, and interpretation to dissect important primitive self and object representations.

A session that opened with the patient saying, "I'm very depressed today," illustrates how depression may emerge as the linking affect in a particular object-relation dyad, and how this depressively tinged dyad may defend against a split-off, aggressively charged object relations dyad. The two main dyads activated in this session are those of a lonely self, depressively longing for closeness to someone who will love her, and an abused and exploited self angrily attacking a selfish, distant victimizer. Depressive themes appeared in the patient's report of depressed mood as well as in her hopelessness, hypochondriasis, and preoccupation with death. The depressive affect was associated with a dream recounted early in this 188th session in the twice-weekly psychodynamic psychotherapy of a divorced mother who lived with her eight-year-old son, Josh. Rick was the name of Josh's father.

PATIENT: I'm very depressed today.

THERAPIST: Hmm.

PATIENT: Josh went away for the weekend, you know. He went to Rick's house.

THERAPIST: Mmm. hmm.

PATIENT: And, uh . . . he doesn't want to go there anymore. Figured that was going to happen, but anyway, he came back yesterday morning. . . . Danny [a friend of the patient's] ended up spending the entire weekend with me. . . . It seems that every time I'm with him, I dream about Larry [a longed-for boyfriend] that night.

THERAPIST: You said you're feeling depressed.

PATIENT: Yeah.

THERAPIST: Wanna tell me about it?

Since no higher-priority defensive themes were present, the therapist focused on the predominant affect in the session at this point.

PATIENT: I'm just feeling (*inaudible*) depressed today, because of the dream.

THERAPIST: What's the dream?

PATIENT: Um, I dreamt that . . . I don't remember the whole thing. I remember looking out the window, and I was sitting . . . my window's by this great big park and, um, he [Larry] was sitting in the park on this bench, and my son was looking out the window too, and then my son went down there, and then I was sitting in my apartment and I was saying, *Oh, should I go down there? Should I walk past?* I was looking in my closets trying to find something to wear to walk past. I was silly, but that's what it was just about, and then I finally did go downstairs, you know, and he waved. I walked past, and I was afraid to acknowledge that he was sitting there, and he waved to me, you know, and like motioned me to come over, and I did, and then we started talking, and then I woke up, my son woke me up. I just felt very depressed (*inaudible*).

The manifest content of the dream contained the object relations dyad:

Insecure Self — *Desiring* — *Longed-for Object (Larry)*

THERAPIST: What struck you about the dream?

PATIENT: I always dream about him when I'm with somebody else, always. I don't know what struck me, I just . . . him happy, acknowledge me to come over and talk to me. See, like when Josh . . . see, Josh is driving me nuts, that's why I asked Rick to take him to his house, you know.

She associated to hostile feeling toward her son and the wish to push him away.

And, um, Saturday morning, when they left, I called Larry at his job, he was working. . . . I said, "There's gonna be nobody here for the whole weekend, do you wanna come over?" And he said no. He said, "I don't want to see you," and he slammed the phone down. He said, "And stop calling me." And then I called him back, and there's this big thing on the phone. He kept hanging up, and I kept calling back. It went on like for an hour and a half, until he finally stopped answering or something. I had this whole fantasy that I was gonna get him to come over, you know. I had it all figured out.

Her next association was to an angry interchange with Larry over his wish to push her away. Notice that two early associations to this rather serene dream contained considerable aggressive affect.

The therapist went on to confront the patient with her wish for an un-available man and her disinterest in Danny, who appeared to be available. This confrontation led the patient to devalue Danny while expressing her contempt for men in general, whom she depicted as self-centered.

[Danny's] like, every bad thing in a male that I cannot stand he has, you know. He's totally obsessed with sports, and he's always watching sports. His whole weekend he spent at my apartment he sat there watching every kind of sports event that came on. I can't stand that. That's one thing . . . I mean, he's into all this stock market crap. . . . He's constantly watching that channel, you know, with all those stock reports on it. He's just too . . . he's boring. And I hate that crap. I hate it. And I'm not attracted to him physically in any way at all, and yet I spent the entire weekend with him, and I had sex with him and everything, and it was horrible.

The patient went on to speak of her feelings about her son over the week-end. She began by talking of missing him and of feeling "flattered" that he had kept calling her hourly to talk to her. As she continued to speak of the calls, however, her tone turned critical: "It was a little annoying because he didn't stop with the phone. He woke me up at seven o'clock in the morning . . . just to tell me about the Ninja Turtle movie. I had to listen to the whole plot of this ridiculous movie." The therapist intervened with a confrontation, pointing out that the patient was dismissive of those who seemed to care about her (Josh and Danny) and longed for an unavailable man. The patient denied the therapist's observation but in so doing provided confirmatory material by speaking of her longings for another man—an unavailable mar-ried man. The therapist pursued the question of why the patient felt com-pelled to invite a man she so detested to spend the weekend with her.

PATIENT: 'Cause I don't want to be alone, I was afraid.

THERAPIST: What were you afraid of?

PATIENT: Because I'm still having all these symptoms, these chest pains and all kinds of crap. I've not been able to catch my breath . . .

THERAPIST: What physical crap?

PATIENT: I get chest pains, and I get shortness of breath, and I get, uh, all sorts of heart-type things. . . . I went out to dinner with my father and my sister. . . . I didn't want to go. . . . I kept imagining the headlines— "Woman Dies of Heart Attack at Table in Restaurant." . . . I'm obsessed with stuff like that. . . . Something's wrong with me, and they haven't found it yet. . . . I'm convinced, I really am, I'm totally convinced. . . . That's why I asked Danny to stay. . . . I feel like I'm manipulating him or something, and then I feel guilty, you know.

The patient responded to the confrontation about seeking out devalued men by retreating into her intense somatic preoccupations and hypochondriacal thinking. The therapist confronted her again, noting that being "afraid of a heart attack any minute certainly provides you with a rationalization [for] having people around you all the time." Here the therapist was confronting the secondary gain of the somatic symptoms (using them to manipulate people into being with her). Note that this intervention is considered a confrontation rather than an interpretation, since the patient was *conscious* of her manipulativeness.

The confrontation was followed by the patient's fantasy that her father had dropped dead: "I called my father Sunday morning. There was nobody there, and I panicked. This goes on constantly. My sisters are getting tired of it. . . . I don't even call them anymore. I panic as soon as he's not there because I think he dropped dead in the apartment."

This fantasy raised the possibility that some of her hypochondriacal fears–specifically, the fear that she was dying–defended against aggression toward her father. The following expression of conscious hostility toward men was consistent with this view.

If I felt physically okay, I probably woulda called Danny and said, "Don't come over." (*pause*) And then I go outside, I went out with Sharon [a friend] . . . and I had more fun with her than with Danny the whole weekend. . . . I said to Sharon last night I'd like to find a hermaphrodite, you know. A woman with male organs. That would be a perfect boyfriend for me. (*chuckle*) I can't stand

men so much. Sometimes I . . . get so angry I . . . I can't explain it. I go nuts. I
don't know why.

We begin to see that although the patient desperately longed for closeness to a man, she did not allow herself this. She chose unavailable or un-
appealing men. We also see that she was intensely angry at men. So her
dilemma was, to put it somewhat starkly, that she longed for closeness to
men but hated them at the same time. There were two conflicting object relations dyads: the dependent, insecure self, trying to entice the idealized
man, and the independent, contemptuous self, attacking worthless men.

What became clearer as the session proceeded were the specific failings of
the bad object, that is, why she experienced such animosity. In this portion of
the session, we see how exploration of the patient's need to relate to either
unavailable men or devalued men was initially defended against with
hypochondriacal rationalizations. Interpretation of this defense led to the
emergence of the feelings of overt hostility toward men. As we discussed in
chapter 1, the entry into awareness of such hostility can be actively defended
against, often by an oscillation in the dyad. Here the patient suddenly
shifted and became the devalued object herself, the recipient of her own hostility. "I don't think I'll ever have a normal relationship with anybody, you
know. I don't think I'm capable of caring about anybody. . . . I think that all
I'm interested in is myself." This is a frequent pattern in depression. The
overt expression of anger toward the devalued other is immediately followed by an interchange of roles. In the session, the patient became the selfish, devalued object that men had been just moments before. Notice also
what the patient criticized in herself–the incapacity to care about others. This
resonates with her earlier descriptions of men as entirely self-absorbed, with
their sports and "stock market crap." This theme would recur.

As the patient attacked this devalued self, a depressive tone reemerged in
the session. "I don't get pleasure out of things that most people do. One
pleasure I get out of . . . I love to drink, I love to eat, and I can't even do that
anymore. I won't even taste anything. . . . I used to read books. . . . I don't
read books anymore." The patient continued to speak of her lack of any
genuine interests and her feelings of alienation.

PATIENT: Well, what are you supposed to do when you're not like other
people? Pretend you are? Is that what you're supposed to do? Like
when you're from another planet.

THERAPIST: You would like the world to meet you at where you're at.

PATIENT: (*chuckle*) That'd be nice.

THERAPIST: And if you need to change yourself in some ways in order to gain a lot of contentment, that enrages you.

The therapist confronted the patient's passivity and entitlement.

PATIENT: Yeah, there's a part of me that has contempt for this other crap.

THERAPIST: What is it that you have contempt for?

The therapist clarified the strong affect.

PATIENT: I don't know. [Whatever is] boring.

THERAPIST: What's boring?

PATIENT: Then why is my sister (*inaudible*).

The feeling of contempt was linked by association to the sister. Based on material from previous sessions, the therapist reminded the patient of how envious she was toward her sister. The patient conceded that she had envied her sister "in ways, yeah, moneywise. . . . Everytime I try to do something wrong, though, it screws up . . . I don't fit in."

The patient next told of going to dinner with her father and sister.

PATIENT: It's like a real cramped restaurant, you know. I don't feel comfortable in places like that. I feel very paranoid, sort of, not paranoid. I feel uncomfortable. Couldn't enjoy the food. . . . I was mad because I couldn't eat this food. . . . I was getting annoyed because they were sitting there talking about the food. I couldn't taste it. . . . And I kept saying something like, "What does it taste like? What does it taste like?" It was horrible. . . . You know, like I said to my father, "I coulda ordered a plate of dog food in here, what's the difference?" It doesn't matter. . . . Well, I felt really upset that I couldn't taste anything, it's horrible.

THERAPIST: Well, clearly people go out to dinner for more reasons than just what the food tastes like.

When the therapist confronted the patient with her avoidance of any of the interpersonal feelings stirred up by dinner with her father and sister, she responded: "No, it makes it interesting because none of us had tasted this kind of food before. . . . And they were sitting there talking about their income tax forms. . . . I've never filled out an income tax form in my life, so that had nothing to do with me, and I couldn't join in that conversation." Again, people were so preoccupied with themselves that they ignored her. With the recurrence of this theme, it began to become apparent that a key attribute of the bad object was that it was self-preoccupied and unable to care for the patient.

The therapist did not choose to articulate this point but rather confronted the patient's hostile passivity: "You use your weaknesses in an aggressive way against people." The therapist then interpreted that the patient's stance of passivity and weakness was in fact a defense against her powerful aggressiveness.

PATIENT: They didn't know I felt uncomfortable.

THERAPIST: You still kept clubbing with the fact that you could not taste. . . . And you were so angry that you don't have what your sisters have . . . and you have a furious rage that keeps you paralyzed. . . . And I think that what you would like to do is to come to me and complain, to tell me how awful things are with you, and the fact that doesn't help you one iota, but the question is, what are you gonna do? How did you let things get so rotten?

The therapist becomes more specific, identifying the rage as envy toward her sisters.

PATIENT: I didn't (*chuckle*) let them get rotten. These things happen to me.

THERAPIST: Yes, but you see what you do. You refuse in a very obstinate way to take responsibility for any of your unhappiness, and it's without reason.

The therapist next tried to show the patient that the same process was taking place in the transference and was undermining the treatment. "It's like therapy at this point: it's not helping you because you can't help people with things that they see as out of their control." The patient continued to protest that she couldn't have advanced because of her emotional problems.

THERAPIST: You're very defensive about it and really refuse to look at yourself now. You want to say, "I'm born this way. I have bad luck. The world is rotten. It's everybody else's fault." And you're stubborn about it.

PATIENT: What am I supposed to do, settle for nothing? Settling for second-best all my life, you know. Sometimes I would rather be down and out—a drug addict—than be stuck in the middle like I am now, you know what I mean? In comparison to my sisters . . . why bother trying, living in a nice apartment . . . and screw it. I'd become a complete derelict or something. What the hell is the difference? I'm stuck in the middle, that's what it feels like. Clawing my way into being a receptionist or something. . . . Why should I hafta work really hard to be a mediocre nothing, you know, I'd rather just be nothing.

The therapist's interpretation of the envious rage led the patient to talk passionately about her resentment about being second-best, confirming the interpretation. As the patient continued, it became clear that her rage was turned destructively and spitefully against her self. There was indeed a triumphant and vengeful quality to her fantasy of becoming a derelict or drug addict.

This session was typical of a prolonged phase of this patient's treatment, which was marked by angry, passive complaints about her sad fate, and illustrates how depression defends against aggressive feelings—in this instance, feelings of envious rage and anger at perceived victimization. By the end of the session, the patient's entitlement and feelings of unjust deprivation became quite explicit, along with her spiteful wishes to sabotage her own life. In this session, the therapist succeeded in bringing these affects directly into awareness. The therapist also made an effort to demonstrate to the patient that her externalizing defenses were undermining the psychotherapeutic work. The patient did little work with this idea in this session. A possible impeding factor at this point in the treatment was unconscious envy of the therapist, a successful woman approximately the patient's own age. It is possible that the patient was sabotaging the treatment out of similar feelings of spiteful envy of the therapist. More active work with the transference in the session—exploring, for example, whether the patient had any feelings toward the therapist that were similar to her envious feeling for her sister—might have greatly expedited the treatment at this point.

The abrupt shifts in the patient's perception of herself and others in the session were, of course, characteristic of the borderline patient. This shift in perception was apparent as she began speaking of her son's multiple phone calls affectionately and then suddenly experienced him as an entitled, demanding burden. It corresponded with the shift from an initial self representation as a desired mother to a subsequent one as an abused and overburdened woman. A devalued introject was projected onto Danny, Josh, and men in general, but then, when the patient's anger became quite conscious, she assumed the role of the devalued object, as someone weird, selfish, unlike normal people and incapable of relationships. Identification with the devalued introject allowed the patient to defend against her intense rage, but at the price of feeling worthless and depressed.

A number of part-self and part-object dyads may be identified in this session:

1. A self (experienced as a deprived and overburdened mother) longing for an idealized romantic male figure (Larry) and feeling sad at his unavailability and the unrequited feelings
2. A devalued, alienated self ("I'm not like other people"; "I'm weird") rejected by the idealized object and feeling enraged
3. A desired self (mother) sought after by a loving son and feeling "flattered"
4. An overburdened, deprived self (mother, daughter, sister) forced to seek the caring and attention of a self-involved other (Danny, Josh, her father) and feeling disgust and contempt
5. An overburdened, deprived self envious and enraged at privileged others (sister, perhaps the therapist)

The first dyad was present in the manifest content of the dream. The feelings of being unwanted by the object were defended against by activation of the third dyad. This could not be sustained as the fourth dyad surfaced, signaled by the perception of the son as demanding and burdensome.

SUICIDALITY IN THE BORDERLINE PATIENT

Suicidal threats, gestures, and overt attempts are commonly encountered in the treatment of borderline patients. The lifetime mortality from suicide among borderline patients has been estimated to be about 10 percent (Stone 1993a; Paris 1993). Suicide threats are verbal or nonverbal communications intended to induce concern in another person that the patient will attempt suicide. They may take the form of direct coercive statements ("If you don't do [this or that] for me, I will kill myself"), or they may be conveyed in more subtle messages veiled in anxiety-generating ambiguity ("The way I've been feeling lately, there's no telling what may happen"). Gestures are overt behaviors that give the appearance of a suicidal intent but are not truly intended to cause death. Of course, patients may die from suicidal gestures gone awry. Finally, borderline patients may engage in self-damaging acts with the intent to cause pain, see blood, or cause damage for its own sake. Such parasuicidal behaviors are not, strictly speaking, suicidal acts, although they may share many of the same psychological determinants.

In dealing with suicidality during the treatment of borderline patients, the therapist needs to assess the acute risk of suicide, diagnose its sources, provide the necessary structure to protect the patient and the treatment, and intervene therapeutically to transform suicidal and parasuicidal intentions into an understanding of their underlying motivations. The suicidal patient activates powerful countertransference reactions in the therapist. The therapist's ability to process these reactions and use them constructively may be the single most important factor in effective work with the suicidal borderline patient.

RISK FACTORS FOR SUICIDE
IN THE BORDERLINE PATIENT

In assessing the suicide risk in a given borderline patient, consideration of a number of risk factors identified in long-term follow-up studies, case series, and clinical practice may offer some guidance. These factors include comorbid conditions and symptoms, social and occupational factors, family and developmental factors, characterological features, and demographic characteristics. Comorbid substance abuse is an important risk factor for suicide. Alcohol, barbiturates, benzodiazepines, opioids, and cocaine all increase the risk. The possibility of suicide is also increased in the presence of a comorbid Axis I affective illness. Among a group of borderline inpatients, Fyer and her colleagues (1988) demonstrated an increased risk of serious suicide attempts when substance abuse or affective disorder accompanied the borderline diagnosis; there was a further and statistically significant increase when substance abuse and affective illness were present together. With borderline patients, as with depressed patients in general, a history of prior suicide attempts is an important risk factor.

A number of social and occupational factors indicate a heightened risk of suicide in borderline patients. The first of these is a chaotic lifestyle. The patient may have no permanent home and be living for brief periods with one friend after another. A poor work history or the inability to sustain an interest in some hobby or pursuit increases the risk (Stone 1993a). Michael Stone has also pointed out that having no (or almost no) friends is a risk factor for borderline patients. Being single and living alone is also a predictor.

Several family and developmental factors contribute to the risk of suicide. A family that is unsupportive or hostile to the treatment should be considered a flag for increased risk. Being an adolescent or young adult and continuing to live with such a family further increases the risk, according to Stone (1993a). A history of significant early childhood losses, such as deaths of significant others, has been shown by Kjelsberg and his colleagues (1991) to increase the risk of suicide. Finally, a developmental history of exposure to repeated intrafamilial traumata, such as incest, physical abuse, or extreme psychological cruelty, constitutes a risk factor (Stone 1993a).

Within the overall borderline organization, a number of specific personality attributes signal added risk. These include schizoid features. The therapist should be particularly cautious when a patient demonstrates an aloofness in the session and does not engage emotionally with him or her. Paranoid personality traits constitute a risk factor when the patient adopts a paranoid stance toward the therapist. Evidence of a chronic lack of concern for the self and others is an ominous sign. Finally, impulsivity, dishonesty, and antisocial features increase the risk of suicide.

Recent studies have identified a number of demographic risk factors among borderline patients. Joel Paris and his colleagues (1989) have reported an increased risk for suicide among the better educated patients in their sample of borderline inpatients. In his follow-up study, Stone (1993a) found that borderline patients between the ages of sixteen and thirty, those with middle-class or higher socioeconomic status, and males had a higher rate of suicide.

DISTINGUISHING CHARACTEROLOGICAL FROM AFFECTIVE SUICIDALITY

Broadly speaking, suicidal ideation in borderline patients has its primary source either in character pathology or affective illness. Of course, these two contributors are not mutually exclusive and are typically found in admixture. The therapist's task is to determine which factor is most prominent at the moment. Different technical approaches apply when suicidality is primarily characterological or primarily affective.

In affective suicidality, the suicidal wishes arise from the unremitting pain of the depression and the associated lack of hope that it will ever cease, or from intense frustration and anger turned inward. Anhedonia makes it difficult for the patient to find any relief. Intense guilt feelings may impel the patient to suicide. In the case of psychotic depression, delusional guilt or other delusional ideas may dictate suicide. In characterological suicidality, on the other hand, suicide or the threat of suicide are called on as solutions to long-standing intrapsychic conflicts. Typically these conflicts are related to anxieties associated with intensely aggressivized internal object relations. Early life experiences such as physical abuse, recurrent or protracted severe physical pain, other traumatic experiences, or constitutional predisposition may contribute to the borderline patient's ultimate internalization of self and other as torturer and victim.

When the patient's aggression is stimulated by current anger, frustration, or envy, self-destruction provides a means to cope with the internalized tormentor. The patient may gratify intense aggressive wishes by physically attacking the self, as an identification with the aggressor. The patient attempts to reverse the experience of self-as-victim by becoming her own torturer. In other situations, the attack on the self represents an attack on internal hated objects. Suicidal behavior is often a means by which the patient exerts control over others, and thus the patient may try to control dangerous and hated internalized objects that have first been projected onto others. In addition to the primary gain that suicidality may provide in coping with aggressive internalized object relations, it may also bring about secondary rewards: attention and concern, the privileges of the sick role, or the control of others to gain specific objectives in the external world. The presence of opportunities for such secondary gain reinforces suicidality. For some patients, characterological suicide becomes a way of life.

Before assuming that the suicidality is primarily characterological, the therapist should carefully assess the nature of the depression, using the criteria described in the first section of this chapter. In the presence of a severe depressive syndrome, suicidality should be assumed to be secondary to the depressive syndrome, and the affective disorder should be actively treated. A number of signs alert the therapist to the likelihood of characterologically based suicidality. First, the presence of one of the personality disorders—especially borderline proper, histrionic, sadomasochistic, infantile, narcissistic, or antisocial—should raise suspicion of a strong characterological component. Second, the finding of a severe suicidal preoccupation in disproportion to the severity of the depression is an indicator of characterological suicidality. Another suggestive finding is a history of preoccupation with suicide or threats of suicide as a prominent theme throughout the patient's life, especially when such preoccupations do not wax and wane with episodes of affective illness. Suicidality that increases specifically in response to interpersonal events is also suggestive of a strong characterological component. Secondary gain from suicidality should also raise the therapist's suspicion of a characterological source. Finally, for some patients suicidality is such a constant theme that it has become woven into their way of life. These patients' principal mode of relating may be as a victim to a life-saver, and they may only be able to form friendships with those willing to enter into such rescue relationships.

Case Example

A woman in her early forties consulted a therapist with the chief complaint, "I've always had thoughts of suicide, but a few weeks ago I reached a turning point where they seemed to make rational sense. I decided that I had nothing to live for, and so I thought I had better see someone." The woman described a chronic mild depression, but she had not been anhedonic, always having been able to obtain pleasure from a number of intellectual pursuits and relationships. Over the past weeks, she reported a temporary difficulty in falling asleep, but she had been able to correct it by adjusting her bedtime. Her appetite had increased recently. She denied any change in concentration, continued to function in a responsible job, and denied anhedonia. No other signs of depression were present. During the initial consultation, her affect appeared only mildly depressed, and she displayed a biting, albeit self-effacing, sense of humor. Although the patient denied any current suicidal intent, the consultant was impressed by the way in which the patient spoke of how she could successfully kill herself. She presented these options in a way that conveyed a sense of great power and made the therapist feel that he was being at once challenged to keep the patient alive and told that there was nothing he could do should she choose to die. The patient spoke of most of the important figures in her life in a condescending manner and was subtly condescending to the consultant as well. She also presented herself as a victim in relationship after relationship in which she was summarily rejected for no apparent reason. The patient's early childhood was characterized by relentless verbal abuse by an alcoholic and controlling mother.

This patient's suicidality appeared to be mainly characterological in origin. It was in disproportion to the degree of depression. It appeared to be used to convey a sense of power and control. It was a chronic feature of the patient's life, even at times when she was only mildly depressed. Finally, it appeared in the context of a narcissistic personality disorder.

TACTICAL APPROACHES TO SUICIDALITY

Since psychosis, substance abuse, and major depression increase risk in a borderline patient with suicidal ideation, the presence of these factors should be ascertained by the therapist. Each should be addressed as it contributes to suicidality. Thus, neuropleptic medication or hospitalization may be called for when the suicidal patient is in a psychotic state. Active substance abuse may need to be addressed by admission into a detoxification program and subsequent rehabilitative treatment. If a major depression is present, concurrent treatment with antidepressant medication, electroconvulsive therapy (ECT), or short-term hospitalization may be indicated.

Once these complicating factors have been addressed, the therapist must determine whether outpatient treatment is safe. The question is whether the patient is willing and able to enter into a contract that protects against suicide, and whether the patient's assurances about such a contract can be trusted. For the contract to be effective, the patient should understand its necessity, and its specific terms should be developed through a mutual process of negotiation. The patient should understand that in committing to outpatient treatment he must ensure that he and the treatment are safeguarded from his self-destructiveness. Treatment cannot work if it can be held hostage to the patient's suicidal wishes.

The therapist explains to the patient that undertaking (or continuing) outpatient treatment is feasible only if the patient can assure the therapist that he will take the measures necessary to ensure that he will not act on suicidal wishes. The therapist invites the patient to collaborate in developing a structure to accomplish this. In doing so, it is important to control any possible secondary gain. A contract that provides, for example, that the patient will call the therapist at any hour of the day or night when feeling suicidal may actually reinforce suicidal preoccupation because it may provide secondary gain in the form of consciously sought contact with the therapist. A customary contract about suicide calls for the patient to speak freely about suicidal feelings in sessions. If the patient has suicidal wishes between sessions, he is expected not to act on them but to speak of these feelings in the next session. If at any point the patient is not sure that he can keep himself from acting on suicidal impulses, he agrees in advance to go to a psychiatric emergency room where the immediate risk may be evaluated.

The negotiation of such a contract is a process (Kernberg et al. 1989; Yeomans, Selzer, and Clarkin 1992). The discussion of the contract is expected to induce anxiety and bring into play many of the patient's characteristic defenses. The therapist does not address these interpretively but simply confronts the patient with the fact that outpatient treatment is not feasible unless safety can be ensured. At the same time, the therapist invites the patient to propose a plan to protect the treatment. In this way, the therapist conveys to the patient that he must share responsibility for the treatment and his own survival. The patient's active involvement in the process is essential. A realistic discussion of the risk of suicide to the treatment and of the patient's responsibility also undercuts a frequently harbored unconscious fantasy that the therapist has omnipotent rescue powers. The therapist should provide the patient with opportunities to discuss his feelings about what is proposed. The therapist should devote just as much attention to a patient's eager compliance with the proposed contract as to any overt resistance to it. Often more than one session is necessary to negotiate the contract. When treatment is already under way and concern about suicidality arises for the first time, the therapist should interrupt all other work to introduce an appropriate contract.

Of course, if the therapist is to rely on the patient's assurance, he must have confidence in the patient's word. To make this judgment, several factors should be considered. Evidence of prior instances of dishonesty, a paranoid stance toward the therapist, the presence of schizoid aloofness, extreme impulsivity, an expressed lack of concern for self, severe anxiety, or the absence of a social support system may call the patient's word into question. In such instances, a period of hospitalization may be necessary.

As the psychotherapy of the borderline patient proceeds, the therapist should be alert to signs of suicidal thinking or threats of suicide. Whenever such themes appear in a session, they must take first priority for intervention. Thus, although the therapist may listen for a while in the session to understand the context and meaning of the suicidal references, obtain further clarification, or lay the groundwork for subsequent interventions, he should reserve adequate time in that session to explore fully the suicidal thoughts and to make the appropriate interventions.

The intervention of choice in psychodynamic psychotherapy for borderline patients is interpretation, and this approach can be safely used when an appropriate contract is in place. The therapist uses clarification, confrontation, and interpretation to explain to the patient the unconscious motivations behind the wish for or threat of suicide. Paying attention to the state of the transference is particularly important here for two reasons. First, particular transference paradigms may interfere with the patient's ability to hear and seriously consider the therapist's interpretations. For example, if the relationship with the therapist is experienced predominantly as a struggle to be in control, this aspect of the transference may need to be interpreted as a precursor to the overall interpretation of the actual function of the suicidal threats; otherwise, the patient may ward off the therapist's words as nothing more than an effort to manipulate him. The second reason it is so crucial to examine the transference is that suicidal wishes arising during an ongoing therapy are frequently a response to particular intense transference reactions. The patient may, for example, see the therapist as a cruel, abandoning figure and react by wishing to punish the therapist by making a suicide attempt, thereby simultaneously attacking the therapist and abandoning him through death, rather than being abandoned. Transference interpretations should therefore be incorporated into the overall interpretive work around the suicidal themes.

If the treatment is progressing and suicidal acting out is limited by maintenance of the treatment contract and active confrontation, the patient's suicidality can be expected to reemerge within the structure of the treatment itself. The patient's self-destructiveness becomes translated into efforts to destroy the treatment, since treatment comes to stand for the patient's chance for survival. The destruction of session time, for example, by long angry silences, empty battles, or substantial lateness is frequently an expression of the patient's suicidality. By focusing on the manner in which the patient's suicidal impulses surface within the session to destroy it, the therapist has an excellent opportunity to analyze suicidality within the transference. When such work is actively carried out, there is often a corresponding decrement in suicidal behavior outside of sessions.

When presenting interpretations, the therapist should carefully attend to the patient's reaction. Confirmatory associations, the emergence of direct anger in the session, a more collaborative working atmosphere in the session, and a reduction of suicidal impulses all suggest that the interpretive approach is productive. Occasionally, however, efforts to interpret suicidality do not decrease its immediacy. In such situations, the therapist reminds the patient of the treatment contract and elicits the patient's agreement to maintain the contract while they continue their work together to understand the suicidal feelings. Infrequently, these approaches are not sufficient, and the therapist needs to shift to a limit-setting stance, which will be analyzed later, to restore technical neutrality. In such a situation, the therapist may intervene directly in the patient's life to ensure his safety. This may take the form of involving significant others or of temporarily hospitalizing the patient. Throughout this phase, the therapist should be careful to defuse any illusion that he is omnipotent and can keep the patient alive regardless of the patient's level of participation in the effort.

Understanding the countertransference is especially important in working with suicidal borderline patients. As issues of life and death come directly into play, the therapist's unresolved feelings about suicide, wishes to be a rescuer, need to be in control, or feelings of inadequacy or powerlessness may become activated. Furthermore, the borderline patient's use of such defenses as omnipotent control and projective identification may induce powerful feelings in the therapist or intensify already existing conflicts. The therapist may feel hate for the patient as he projects his own sadism and simultaneously provokes these feelings in the therapist. Hate in the countertransference is an important complication in the treatment of suicidal patients (Maltsberger and Buie 1974). Alternatively, the patient's hopelessness and powerlessness may be activated in the therapist, and he may become paralyzed into inaction. It is when such countertransference feelings are unconscious that they are most apt to influence the therapist's actions. It is helpful for the therapist to pay attention to his fantasies and feeling states, particularly those that seem uncharacteristic or excessive. Consultation with a colleague may be invaluable. Awareness of the counter-transference will aid the therapist in avoiding counterproductive enactments and may help him to identify the self-object dyad activated in the treatment at the moment. This knowledge will aid the therapist in formulating his interpretive interventions around the suicidal themes.

CHAPTER 9

Trauma, Sexual Pathology, and Acting Out

Early childhood trauma of a severe and ongoing nature is so frequent in the histories of borderline patients as to require us to integrate what is known about the sequelae of trauma with observations of borderline patients and with theories about the psychological underpinnings of their behavior. Patients with histories of childhood trauma often present particular dilemmas for psychodynamic treatment. Premature focus on traumatic memories can have a retraumatizing effect, self-destructive urges can be very powerful and erupt suddenly, and early trauma experiences may cause enduring neu robiological dysregulations. This chapter reviews the ways in which childhood trauma shapes adult relationship patterns and the transference and addresses special considerations in conducting TFP with these patients.

Following Judith Herman (Perry and Herman 1993), we conceive of trauma, for the purposes of this chapter, as events (such as severe neglect, physical assault, or sexual victimization, particularly by parents) that would be expected to be traumatic for anyone, thus excluding events that are traumatic by virtue of their idiosyncratic meaning to a particular individual. By this definition, trauma occurs in the childhood and adolescence of a very high proportion (81 percent) of patients diagnosed as borderline (Herman, Perry, and van der Kolk 1989). Comparison between borderline and similarly impaired but nonborderline children has revealed a higher prevalence of parental neglect, sexual and physical abuse, parental criminality, and substance abuse, and significantly more foster placements in the borderline group (Gudzer et al. 1991). Borderline pathology is not an inevitable result of childhood trauma. Estimates of the prevalence of childhood sexual abuse among normal subjects range from 10 to 50 percent (Sachsse 1995), while childhood physical abuse ranges from 6 to 20 percent in the normal population, according to Sachsse's survey of the literature. The particular trauma of parent-daughter incest is two to four times more frequent among borderline patients than in the general population (Stone 1993b).

THE SEQUELAE OF CHILDHOOD TRAUMA

Severe, prolonged psychological and physical traumata during childhood and adolescence have an array of sequelae extending beyond the post-traumatic stress syndrome characteristic of adult survivors of comparatively circumscribed traumatic events such as rape, combat, or disaster. The particular modes of coping developed in response to ongoing trauma render the individual vulnerable to further harm, through self-inflicted injury, victimization by others, and seemingly uncontrollable misfortune. Complex unconscious mechanisms falling under the category of repetition compulsion lead these patients to induce in the environment new editions of the original traumatic experiences.

The symptoms with which survivors of severe and prolonged trauma during childhood present themselves for psychotherapy include insomnia, sexual dysfunction, experiences of derealization and depersonalization, pervasive anger, persistent wishes to die or be killed, self-mutilation, substance abuse, and suicide attempts. The clinical presentation is diffuse and complex, with disturbances in interpersonal relationships and in the sense of personal identity. Some chronically traumatized people are beset by anxieties about their bodies, reacting with exaggerated concern to what others would regard as minor ailments and discomforts and experiencing a sense of conviction that something is radically wrong with various organ systems. Others exhibit profound denial of bodily concerns and neglect their physical health. Still others present a combination of somatic anxiety and denial. Many chronically traumatized individuals are hypervigilant, anxious, and agitated, while others live in a numbed and dissociated state that puts them at chronic risk of harm. Most are plagued by the nightmares, flashbacks, and startle reactions typical of post-traumatic stress disorder. These shared features have led some clinicians to equate PTSD with borderline pathology and to reason backward from the latter to an assumption of early trauma, sometimes with deleterious clinical consequences.

Over time the sequelae of severe childhood trauma come to include such psychosomatic symptoms as tension headaches, gastrointestinal disturbances and abdominal, pelvic, and back pain, tremors, choking sensations, and nausea (Herman 1993). These symptoms tend to increase over time. In contrast to and often coexistent with symptoms of hyperreactivity, it is not uncommon for traumatized patients to present with analgesia, as measured by the ability to tolerate the immersion of their hands in ice water for prolonged periods. A striking example was a patient who tolerated dental extractions without anesthesia and who walked for some miles with a broken ankle, which she finally noticed only because it became swollen. One may postulate that pain evokes dissociative phenomena in such patients.

Prisoners during captivity as well as chronically abused children learn to exploit their capacities for trance, denial, minimization, thought suppression, and dissociation in order to endure distress (Russell 1989; Shengold 1989). The extent of dissociative symptoms in borderline patients may be linked to the severity of childhood abuse (Herman et al. 1989).

Intractable depression is the most common finding in studies of chronically traumatized people. That medication rarely results in symptomatic relief in these cases is understandable when their depression is recognized as stemming from multiple sources. The exhaustion resulting from chronic sleeplessness and hyperarousal; the shame over the impaired functioning due to concentration difficulties imposed by dissociation; the debased self-concept, paralysis of initiative, and damaged relationships of the chronically traumatized person, all contribute to the picture of depression, as does the ongoing influence of unexpressed rage (Herman et al. 1989).

The psychobiological response to trauma may be short-lived in the case of a single traumatic event if it is promptly and adequately treated. In cases of severe, ongoing trauma for which treatment is delayed, or which occurred before its verbal processing was possible, psychobiological sequelae may extend over many years. In either case, the typical response is bimodal: hyperactivity, hyperarousal, and hypermnesia alternating or simultaneous with psychic numbing, avoidance, amnesia, and anhedonia (van der Kolk 1987). This bimodal response may contribute to an inner sense of fragmentation that is often projected and enacted when the patient creates chaotic scenarios. Traumatized patients may express the bimodal response through seemingly paradoxical behavior, such as combining excessive fears of pain with seeking opportunities for serious injury. The paradox becomes understandable when its psychological meaning is explored. The exaggerated fear of pain or of medical procedures represents the expectation of re-experiencing the original trauma, of being again helpless, terrified, and injured. Such fears may also represent hyperarousal in the service of preparing the ego for assault, assuring that one is never caught to be off guard. Seeking reinjury represents an unconscious attempt to master the trauma through denial or to identify oneself with the victimizer, with one's own body as the victim. By being the active agent rather than the passive victim of trauma, the patient maintains a sense of being in control. Underlying each aspect of the paradoxical behavior is a fantasy based on an unconscious object relationship.

CASE EXAMPLES

Ms. L., raped and battered by her father from the age of four, displayed marked distress over several weeks about the pain of a sprained wrist. At the same time, she experienced impulses to reinjure her wrist and played volleyball without the recommended brace, against the remonstrances of friends. Afterward she showed her doctor how the injured wrist had once again become swollen and painful, seeking comfort and sympathy for the injury she herself had inflicted. These enactments reflected identification with the batterer and at the same time relief of the sense of passive victimization through being able to blame herself for the damaged wrist, while simultaneously generating feelings of helplessness in her doctor.

Our current understanding of the biological effects of trauma include extreme autonomic responses and increased endogenous opioid output in response to stimuli reminiscent of the trauma; decreased serotonin activity (linked with aggressiveness and impulsivity); decreased glucocorticoid reaction to stress; and traumatic nightmares in stages II and III of sleep. Recent studies of maltreated children indicate hypothalamic-pituitary-adrenal axis dysregulation, increased catecholamines, decreased hippocampal volume, altered growth and physical development, and immune system dysfunction (Putnam and Trickett 1997). That the effects of trauma persist and even intensify over time is to some extent explained by retraumatizing life events and by the effects of the repetitive intrusive symptoms—the memories of the trauma, nightmares, flashbacks—which themselves act like repeated traumata by producing hyperarousal.

Borderline patients tend to be hyperreactive to their environment, with hypersensitivity in interpersonal situations. This hypersensitivity may be most closely related to a history of childhood sexual and/or physical trauma and may be mediated through noradrenergic mechanisms (Figueroa and Silk 1997).

Patients who have experienced severe childhood trauma have been described by many observers as exceptionally prone to being abused by others in adulthood. Such patients, lacking the childhood experience of success in defending themselves, and indeed, being unaware of having the right to do so, display an extraordinary proneness to being exploited and mistreated. Learned passivity, ignorance, and lack of social sophistication and skill do not account for this entirely. Traumatized patients experience feelings of worthlessness that find expression in feeling not entitled to defend themselves. Furthermore, they may be willing to undergo humiliating experiences in order to validate their view of the world as cruel and corrupt. They often believe that any kindness from another carries with it the obligation of repayment with sexual submission. Such attitudes are among the determinants of the susceptibility of these patients to repetitions of trauma in adulthood. Many experience a pervasive sense of the imminence of being injured and provoke attack to relieve that anxious anticipation.

Trauma affects memory in complex ways. It interferes with the storage of explicit, semantic memory, that is, memory of sequential events describable in words, with reference to specific time and place, and to the relationships and meanings of the events. On the other hand, trauma enhances the storage of implicit memory, the nonverbal memory manifest in skills, images, habits, emotional associations, and conditioned and sensorimotor responses (van der Kolk 1987; van der Kolk and Fisler 1994). A common example is the patient who is unable to give a coherent narrative account of her life story (impairment of semantic memory) but who is subject to vivid flashbacks that include the reexperiencing of terror and pain (implicit memory) that she is hard put to describe in words.

Like many incest victims, Ms. L. doubted the veridicality of her memories of early childhood sexual abuse; these memories retained a vague, dreamlike quality. In art therapy, she "found herself" drawing scenes that made her vague memories explicit. She reacted with extreme distress to what she experienced as incontrovertible evidence of the accuracy of memories she preferred to doubt. At the same time, she reported nightmares that she "knew" replicated actual experiences of violence and that were followed, upon awakening, by severe pain identical to that inflicted on her in the dream.

The effects of prolonged trauma on memory systems may contribute to the apparent impairment of borderline patients' ability to learn from experience. Furthermore, clinicians as well as family members are often puzzled by the abrupt onset of severe symptoms in patients who have functioned competently for years, apparently dismissing their memories of trauma. Lawrence Kolb (1987) has postulated that in cases of delayed post-traumatic stress disorder, indelible subcortical emotional responses are prevented, by cortical and septohippocampal inhibitory activity, from being activated. Eventually these controls are worn down by aging, drugs, alcohol, or retraumatization: then a delayed post-traumatic response emerges, with physical symptoms and affect states that represent the unmodified somatic memory. A major depressive episode may herald or precipitate the onset of such severe symptoms, and psychotherapy itself can constitute a new and sometimes unmanageable trauma if the evocation of painful memories is carried out too rapidly and without the concomitant shoring up of ego capacities.

Ms. M. obtained a postgraduate degree in history and was about to embark on her career as a teacher when she was beset by vivid memories of the suicide of her brother some years previously. Hospitalized in a suicidal state, she told her therapist at length and in detail the story of being neglected and beaten by a psychotic mother and sexually abused by her father throughout her childhood. As if overstimulated and retraumatized by the reactivation of these memories, she took to her bed, attempting to remain asleep for as many hours of the day as possible. She remained intractably suicidal for over a year despite attempts at treatment with medication. Electroshock therapy was eventually recommended, but like many traumatized patients, she refused on the grounds that she feared being unconscious and perhaps dying: she wanted to be in control of her own death, not taken by surprise by death at the hands of another person.

Ms. R. functioned capably as a mother, homemaker, community leader, and nurse until the death of one of her children. She became depressed and was hospitalized. In the hospital, the physician became interested in her case and provided daily psychotherapy sessions during which her history of severe sexual abuse by an incestuous father and uncle, not forgotten but suppressed until now, was elicited. The patient was encouraged to relive her painful experiences and soon experienced dissociated states in which she had different names. At the same time, Ms. R. deteriorated into a state of implacable self-destructiveness and developed the conviction that she was intrinsically evil. "These terrible things would not have happened to me," she said, "if I had not been an evil child." Intensive encouragement to reveal the humiliating and rage-infused details of her childhood experience constituted a retraumatization that overwhelmed her previously effective, if fragile, defenses.

These cases illustrate the importance of pacing in psychotherapy. The exposure of traumatic memories without first assessing and, where necessary, bolstering the patient's ego strength can be harmful. In patients who have experienced the emotional and physical neglect that often accompany sexual and physical abuse, the kindly interest of the therapist can fulfill long-suppressed needs for attention and concern. The gratification of these needs serves as a motive to produce more traumatic memories, which in turn stimulate increasingly desperate efforts at defense: dissociation, self-inflicted injuries, and regression into psychosis.

Superimposed upon and entangled with the biological effects of trauma is the psychology of rage, a primary affect activated by frustration or pain (Kernberg 1994). Its earliest function can be seen as the elimination of a source of distress or of an obstacle to gratification: its aim is the removal or destruction of a "bad object." When the capacity for intersubjectivity has developed, the aim of rage is to make the object suffer: hatred becomes possible, along with sadism, the fusing of aggression with pleasure. As a child develops defenses against sadism, pleasurable fantasies of injuring or killing others may be projected and then experienced as a need to dominate and control a threatening other in order to avoid being injured, tormented, or killed.

The internalization of a relationship with a desired and needed object who causes pain and frustration and is thus hated results in unconscious identification with both the powerful, teasing, withholding, sadistic object and the frustrated, injured, terrified victim. This unconscious identification with both victim and victimizer intensifies the actual relationship with the traumatizing object out of a need to control or punish the victimizer or to influence a bad object to become transformed into a good one (Kernberg 1994). The result is counterphobic enactments in which the patient provokes a known victimizer to injure her once again.

Ms. L. enacted her identification with victim and victimizer in a variety of ways. With respect to her sprained wrist, it emerged that reinjuring it represented a repetition of a critical interaction with her father when, having injured her arm in a bicycle accident, she complained of pain: the father struck her arm and fractured it. "Now you have something real to complain about," he said. In reinjuring her wrist, she enacted identification both with the sadistic father and with the hurt child.

She described the father's smiling teasing, and the family's pervasive apprehensiveness as to when this teasing would shift into violence. Meanwhile, she herself maintained a provocative, smiling manner, proclaiming enigmatically that she would handle "whatever might happen." "What might happen" included the possibility of being struck by a car: one of her favorite games was to see how close she could come to being struck by a car in traffic. Her teasing manner instilled a tense state of anger and anxiety in anyone attempting to make judgments about her safety. This state was a repetition of her own apprehensiveness in response to her father's teasing. And though she brushed off any manifestation of concern with, "I'll take care of it," she was prone to feeling neglected. While proclaiming that she didn't need anyone's help, she experienced her would-be helpers as callous and uncaring.

Ms. L.'s hatred of her father remained disavowed: "I guess I'm afraid to hate him because I always think that one day he will stop hurting me and love me." She projected hatred onto others, experiencing them as hating her, and herself as deserving nothing but to be hated and rejected by others. In countless ways, she contrived to be hurt, betrayed, disappointed, and rejected by a therapist who in fact remained warmly interested in her. Ms. L. was aware of a wish to provoke the therapist's hatred in order to feel secure in a familiar situation, experiencing extreme tension whenever she felt the therapist's intentions to be kindly and genuine. A state of trust and dependence activated memories of feeling similar comfort with her father, only to have her security shattered by a sadistic outburst. Safety involved constant vigilance and conscious efforts to quell wishes to rely on others.

To defend herself against the hazards of human relatedness, she literally blocked out awareness of the feelings of others: she was unaware of the emotional impact her provocativeness had on others. She was genuinely puzzled and nonplussed when asked whether she thought about how a driver would feel if his car struck her during one of her reckless games.

Ms. L. lived with intense anxiety by day and violent nightmares at night. She saw death as promising relief of her distress and remembered longingly the occasions when she had overdosed to the point of unconsciousness. Only the threat of the treatment being broken off prompted her to fight off urges to do so again to gain temporary surcease. Hers was a reality pervaded by hatred of her abuser that was maintained outside awareness. Her efforts to block out that reality included self-mutilation, compulsive risk-taking, abuse of drugs and alcohol, and periods of mutism. (A reality not described in words, either aloud or in thought, seemed to her less real.) She displaced her own suppressed rage onto a faceless driver who could run her down, while her anxiety was transformed into an exhilarating thrill in a primitive reversal of affects.

When a parent repeatedly injures a child, it is often in a context of generalized family violence involving siblings, pets, and the other parent. The rage of the injured child is complicated by affection; sexual wishes; rivalry with siblings and feelings of being special; fears of abandonment and retaliation; concern for the safety of other family members; shame and guilt over being unable to protect them; envy of siblings spared of abuse; and a pervasive sense of being intrinsically bad. In cases of father/stepfather–daughter incest, chronic anger is mixed with guilt that has among its sources the excitement associated with being chosen by the father and triumphing over the mother; rage at a mother who, while failing to protect the child, is often also being battered and terrorized; and the child's own inability to protect the other siblings from incest. These feelings of guilt are compounded by shame that is often explicitly instilled by the parent. Rage, suppressed in the face of these complications, takes the form of chronic irritability, depression, and anxiety.

Ms. A. finally confided in a teacher after years of beatings and sexual assaults by an alcoholic father. When the teacher advised her to escape from her violent family, she found herself unable to do so: were she to leave her mother to endure the father's battering alone, Ms. A. would feel so guilty over abandoning her (even though she could not protect her) that she would feel obliged to kill herself.

Cross-generational incest prevents the integration of parental prohibitions and punishments and rewards into a reliable system of moral and ethical values, leaving the child to be guided by superego structures that are both cruel and lax: the child experiences the world as morally chaotic and unpredictable, and herself as intrinsically bad. These views are often rein-forced explicitly by the traumatizing adult. Unable to make accurate judg-ments regarding the parent's behavior, the child cannot work through the sexually traumatic experience toward a coherent sense of self and a firm as-signment of responsibility to the exploitive adult. Instead, these patients rigidly maintain mutually contradictory internalized object relations in the service of conserving whatever "good" aspects of the incestuous object can be retained, while holding off the traumatic aspects: splitting and identity diffusion protect against the intolerable anxiety of living in a state of hatred, danger, and chaos.

The father of Ms. F. terrorized his wife and ten children for more than a decade. Ms. F. escaped the traumatic household by marrying at eighteen, raised her two children, and did not succumb to depression and dissociated states until the age of forty-five. At this point, following an automobile acci-dent, she developed intractable back pain that required many physical ex-aminations. She experienced these as intolerably intrusive and humiliating, although she did not connect this reaction to her childhood experiences. She became depressed and began to experience "blackouts" during which fam-ily members could not make contact with her. In the course of treatment, she struggled to maintain the view that her depression was a chemical disorder and that the past was irrelevant to her current symptoms, even though these included flashbacks to scenes of childhood violence.

Estranged from the incestuous father for years, Ms. F. felt compelled to visit him on his deathbed. At this time, she expressed the conviction that "Papa" had been a handsome, gallant, loving man to whom she was a spe-cial daughter, while "Daddy" was a cruel brute who had ruined the lives of all the family.

By means of splitting her internal representation of her father, Ms. F. was able to maintain her attachment to fragments of positive experience and to fantasies of him as loving. Rejection of her father as a brute would have left Ms. F. with a rage so intense that she feared it would destroy her.

SELF-MUTILATION IN TRAUMATIZED PATIENTS

The behavioral responses to physical and sexual trauma are multiply deter-mined and express diverse motives. Many patients discover that they can produce significant (if fleeting) mood elevation and decreased dissociation by injuring themselves. Dissociative symptoms seem to be related to insensitivity to pain (Kemperman, Russ, and Shearin 1997). Biological hypotheses have emphasized the impulsive and aggressive aspects of self-injurious behavior, implicating central serotonergic dysfunction (Gardner, Lucas, and Cowdry 1990). Self-mutilation is thought to stimulate production of endorphins so as to provide a momentary euphoria (Coid, Allolio, and Rees 1983), which may contribute to the addictive quality of self-mutilation. It is possible to postulate a role for a substance-P antagonist, a compound recently found to have antidepressant effects, in the euphoric response to self-mutilation.

Self-mutilation can serve as a means to disrupt an unbearable sense of emptiness, of "feeling dead inside," which may either express the identity diffusion of these patients or represent the loss of a previously split-off internal object as a consequence of psychotherapy. Thus, an unexpected outburst of self-injury may occur when a patient becomes conscious of justified anger and hatred toward a remembered abuser without concomitant mourning for the loss of an internal relationship, however painful it may have been. For patients who experience self-injury as painful, it serves as punishment of the self, and sometimes as punishment of a part of the self seen as "bad" by another self-fragment identified with a "good" but punitive parent; the mutilation can serve as a reproach and as vengeance in the context of transference to a therapist seen as rejecting. For some patients, the urge to mutilate parts of the body expresses a fantasy that their self-injury protects someone else against violence (a Christ fantasy) or that a token wound will be accepted in lieu of suicide by an internalized object demanding death as punishment for the disloyalty of exposing the behavior of the abuser in therapy: "Don't tell anyone" is a common component of the sexual abuse of children by adults.

Many of these patients explicitly want to excise or mutilate their breasts or genitals as the source of forbidden excitement or as the aspect of themselves that attracts the abuser.

Trauma in Relation to Eating Disorders

Eating disorders are common among patients who were sexually abused in childhood. Patterns of intense overeating in an attempt at self-soothing may alternate with induced vomiting and purging in response to feelings of self-loathing. Obesity as a form of destruction of sexual attractiveness is very common among victims of incest; weight reduction stirs intense anxiety in these patients. Symptoms of choking or of revulsion toward food or liquids are often reflections of early oral sexual assaults or of punishments involving force-feeding or starvation in childhood.

DISTURBANCES OF THE
SEXUAL LIVES OF TRAUMATIZED PATIENTS

A broad range of sexual pathology is characteristic of patients who have experienced sexual abuse in childhood and adolescence. Impulsive sexual behavior and promiscuity may give the diagnostician a false impression of the patient's capacity for sexual pleasure. Genuine sexual enjoyment is rare among these patients, and even when that capacity is preserved, love relationships are characteristically chaotic. Sexual anesthesia as well as states of uncomfortable sexual overstimulation are common sequelae of childhood sexual abuse. Sexual anesthesia may be associated with promiscuity in the service of denial of emotional meaning of the sexual relationship, or of identification with the abuser of childhood who was seen as cold and unfeeling. Many of these patients have a powerful aversion to being touched; paradoxically, some of these same patients provoke violent attacks that they experience as confirmation of their view of the world as unsafe and hostile. The theme of prostitution is prevalent in the psychotherapy of patients who have experienced incest.

Ms. D. had a father whose gifts always carried with them the demand for sexual repayment. Ms. D. looked with apprehension on such mundane acts of kindness as the therapist's offer to change an appointment for her convenience, linking such actions with her father's expectation of being "paid back." It was only after this issue had been addressed over several years in therapy that Ms. D. was able to request and accept a favor from a friend, or an accommodation from the therapist.

A "friend" gave money to Ms. B. and took her out to dinner from time to time. She made no effort to defend herself against his unwanted sexual advances because she had accepted his gifts. After experiencing herself as having been raped by him, she reacted later with profound anxiety, revulsion, and shame but insisted that she "had to pay back."

Ms. A. had been raped repeatedly by her father from age three until seventeen. In her adolescence, she began to experience orgasm, which greatly compounded her shame and disgust. At the same time, her father began to reward her financially according to how well she "performed." Among the multiple factors that held her back from resuming her once successful scientific career was the fantasy that getting paid for work equated one with a prostitute. At some level, she saw all working people, including her therapist, as selling themselves. This view protected her from painfully envious feelings toward those who lived a productive life and gave her an illusion of moral superiority in the face of her profoundly debased view of herself.

A characteristic submissiveness and sense of being doomed to mistreatment coexist in some of these patients with an underlying vengeful, cynical intention to "prove" the fundamental depravity of others who come to represent the original traumatizer. The experience of repeated sexual abuse, especially when combined with violence, is associated with a state of perpetual apprehensiveness. By placing themselves in dangerous situations and submitting to rape in adulthood, many of these patients find a way of bringing about what they feel is inevitable and thus ending the painful suspense that is linked to their sense of the self as damaged, wicked, and doomed.

The extent to which sexuality has been welcomed and enjoyed may have important prognostic and diagnostic implications. Borderline patients who have a capacity for sexual pleasure tend to respond more favorably to psychotherapy. In cases of sexual anesthesia or discomfort, it is important to differentiate dissociation or extreme repression from other possible causes. Patients who completely lack the capacity for sexual enjoyment, whose lives are devoid of any sexual activity, fantasies, or wishes, may well be those most impaired and most difficult to treat. Severe sexual disturbances can contribute to binge eating as a means of obtaining pleasure while also fending off potential sexual partners by maintaining obesity.

TREATMENT IMPLICATIONS

Isolated traumatic experiences in adulthood may or may not lead to PTSD, but these experiences have little effect on the personality as a whole. By contrast, chronic, repetitive trauma in early childhood and adolescence not only evokes symptoms of stress but also tends to contribute heavily to the development of personality disorders of varying degrees of severity as the array of defenses mustered by the traumatized child to cope with the pervasive physiological and interpersonal sequelae of stress become increasingly maladaptive. A viable treatment plan depends on thorough psychiatric evaluation that encompasses all aspects of the patient's life and leads to a comprehensive diagnostic formulation. But because the defining sequelae of severe trauma represent the implicit and unintegrated somatic, affective, and behavioral memories of the trauma, and because impairment of explicit semantic memory in many patients is intensified by repression, denial, and efforts to suppress and dismiss the painful facts of their lives, diagnostic understanding is often very difficult to achieve until treatment is well established, as illustrated by the following case.

Ms. W., a married, self-reliant, successful businesswoman of Asian origin and the mother of a three-year-old, had been left with her grandmother at age six months so that her parents could pursue their professional careers abroad. She was about a year old when she nearly died of a severe infection and was then given into the care of her other grandmother, who lived in better circumstances but who physically abused the child. Over the ensuing years, the mother of Ms. W. appeared periodically to deposit another baby with the abusive grandmother. Ms. W. became the caretaker and protector of these younger siblings and meanwhile was sexually molested by an alcoholic uncle. Eventually she was reunited with her parents in a remote country, but this rescue had the quality of yet another disruption in the long series of traumata that had been her life: her parents were strangers, her grandmother having been the only mother she ever knew.

She sought treatment because of "rage attacks." In initial interviews, the clinician could not but be struck by how well she had managed in the face of extreme deprivations and stresses. When asked about self-injurious behavior, she denied it, but several months into psychotherapy she let slip the information that she used to overdose in adolescence. She was then able to acknowledge the extent of the "rage attacks," which took the form of hitting herself and banging her head so uncontrollably that her husband had to restrain her to prevent injury. She related all this with a dismissive demeanor: "I did not go into all the details because it's not important."

Treating the trauma instead of the patient can have serious consequences, as the following case illustrates.

Ms. O.'s life was plagued by her parasitic behavior. A talented artist, she depended for financial support on men she despised. Her life passed her by as she failed to use her creative endowment. Her father had been a bigamist who ended up in jail. Her mother, sliding into shame and depression, eventually remarried. The new husband turned out to be a voyeur, peeping at his stepdaughter. This interest was the first attention she felt she had received. In adulthood, she sought out a succession of therapies in which she successfully used her childhood memories of neglect and victimization as a defense against self-reflection ("How else would you expect me, as an abused child, to behave and react?") and as justification for her sense of entitlement. It was not until her midfifties, when she engaged in a treatment that focused on this stance in the transference, that she finally revealed her violent rage and its enactment in stabbing a man in the heat of an argument and attempting to poison her stepfather. It was at that point that she began to move out of her seemingly solidified victim role.

Although some patients who have experienced severe childhood abuse exploit their victimhood, as Ms. O. did, it is more typical for explicit memories of trauma to emerge gradually against marked resistance over the course of months or years of treatment. Because abuse by a parent is typically associated with feelings on the child's part of being responsible for the parent's attacks, acknowledging memories of these experiences is a painful and shame-laden experience. Considerable groundwork must be laid in psychotherapy before it is safe or useful to connect current symptoms with the traumatic memories: these patients typically "know" the origins of their symptoms while lacking the ego strength to tolerate that knowledge.

The basic principle of treatment of traumatized patients is that of building ego strength through the development of a trustworthy therapeutic relationship prior to encouraging retrieval of traumatic memories. The first steps in developing a working relationship consist of establishing a safe and predictable environment in which to carry out the treatment, beginning with arriving at an agreement with the patient as to the difficulties she wants to address in therapy and the problems she foresees in doing this (Yeomans, Selzer, and Clarkin 1992). Thus, the patient's role as agent rather than as victim in the treatment relationship is established from the outset.

Discussing the conditions of therapy in detail and securing the patient's acceptance of the conditions that will make treatment possible (setting the contract) begins to identify the therapy situation as safe and predictable and suggests to the patient that she is not a powerless victim but has control over her life. Suicidal and self-destructive behavior not only serves as a regulator of intolerable affect but also as a means of controlling the environment, to the detriment of the patient, the environment, and the treatment. When the contract-setting process includes explicit plans for how the patient will keep herself safe and healthy, it tends to remove some of the secondary gain of being watched over by a worried doctor who can be injured and undermined by "failure" to protect the patient.

Various special conditions may need to be met if psychotherapy is to take place with traumatized patients: for instance, medication, intensive training in stress management, counseling the family, or providing vocational assistance and advice. A therapist who attempts to undertake all of these tasks and roles is likely so to dilute therapy with survival issues as to render treatment ineffective. These patients are often so severely compromised and live in such constant danger at the hands of others as well as themselves that they have been likened to severe burn cases. As such, they require a treatment team of pharmacologist, social worker, case manager or vocational therapist, internist, and therapist.

Medication is often necessary as an early and sometimes ongoing aspect of the psychotherapy of traumatized patients. Effective psychotherapy cannot be carried out with a severely sleep-deprived patient, nor in the presence of unalleviated depression, flashbacks, or dissociated states. Most therapists engaged in intensive psychotherapy with these patients find it helpful to establish a working relationship with a colleague who prescribes medication, maintains general medical oversight of the case, and provides coverage in the therapist's absence. Such an arrangement guarantees the necessary close observation, provides each colleague with the consultation of the other, and ensures that, in the absence of one doctor, the other is familiar with the case.

Once a workable treatment regimen has been established, the structure of the psychotherapy facilitates the expression of feelings in the transference rather than through somatization or acting out. The therapist's pervasive attitude of neutrality conveys the capacity to register whatever the patient has to say without being overwhelmed by shock, horror, or sympathy. This objective attitude, when the patient identifies with it, strengthens her capacity to tolerate and eventually integrate the remembered trauma and the rage associated with it.

It is important to evaluate the patient's sexual functioning fully in the course of psychotherapy, at the appropriate time. This is often avoided out of the therapist's fear of disturbing the patient—an attitude akin to fear of inquiring about suicidal thoughts lest one "put ideas into the patient's head."

The feelings expressed or disavowed in the transference are typically related to the victim-victimizer paradigm that dominates the inner life of many of these patients. A therapist must be alert to the role being assigned to him in each interaction with the patient (as in any expressive psychotherapy), paying particular attention to the likelihood of being cast in one of these two roles. A second paradigm, that of seducer-seducee, is equally prevalent in the interpersonal landscape inhabited by patient and therapist when childhood seduction has occurred. A tactful yet matter-of-fact acknowledgment of the patient's fears and wishes to be seduced in the here and now helps temper the emotional climate and relieve the patient's anxiety. Meanwhile, it is unwise to speculate as to the motives and feelings of seducer and seducee in the there and then. Considerable damage was done, for example, to a patient and to the therapeutic alliance when the therapist, in response to the patient's distressed recollections of her father's sexual advances, remarked on "how seductive a little girl of four can be." Such confirmation of the patient's irrational belief that her own lustfulness brought about the seduction by an adult did no service to her efforts to sort out the guilt feelings that had pervaded her adult life.

It is only after conditions of safety have been securely established (often over months or even years) that the usual task of psychotherapy, to help the patient develop a coherent life story, can be undertaken. For some traumatized patients, retrieving memories and integrating them into their understanding of themselves are useful, if at all, only at a late stage of the treatment. When patients can tolerate it, the development of a coherent narrative becomes a means of mastering the chronic state of fragmentation and overstimulation that led them to seek treatment.

Although the mechanism by which telling the story brings about symptom relief is not entirely clear, the phenomenon is so common in everyday life as to be taken for granted—hence the tendency of many therapists to encourage the patient to recite traumatic memories at an early stage of treatment. Healthy people who have been even mildly traumatized have a seemingly inordinate need to recount the story again and again until the need eventually fades; then it is as if the trauma has been "metabolized"—incorporated into the person's life history, with an associated modification (however slight) of the person's sense of identity. In telling the story of the near miss, the auto accident, the operation, or the fire in the kitchen, the speaker expects the listener to identify with him. As the listener implicitly fulfills this expectation, the speaker experiences the sympathy, respect, or righteous indignation of the listener with regard to the traumatic experience, and these responses help to shape a new sense of self in the speaker—

as one deserving of compassion, or a hero, or a lucky survivor, or one un-justly treated. The altered sense of self helps compensate for the feelings of helplessness, weakness, and shame that are evoked by threats to life and bodily integrity and thus contributes to recovery from the effects of the trauma. In such cases, the trauma is often incorporated into the person's running autobiography as a positive experience that made him a stronger or more empathic or more optimistic individual. This normal process is a late development in the psychotherapy of traumatized borderline patients (van der Kolk, McFarlane, and Weisaeth 1996).

DANGERS OF RELAPSE AND NEGATIVE THERAPEUTIC REACTIONS

To be freed of long-standing emotional pain and to become capable of func-tioning effectively can have conscious and unconscious negative connota-tions. These include rising expectations from within and without; disappointment that life can never make up for what happened; loss of jus-tification for receiving care; and a fear that getting well invalidates the orig-inal trauma. Giving up illness may mean renouncing revenge and denying the seriousness of childhood (if not lifelong) misery. Paradoxically, vivid nightmares and flashbacks may be the only reliable companions, the only "family" one has: without them, a patient may feel eerily alone. The de-structive impact on the therapist of embittered and paranoid reactions un-leashed by the experience of change for the better can be mitigated by recognition of the meaningfulness and legitimacy of such reactions and by a systematic focus on the negative meanings of progress toward health (Ap-pelbaum, 1996; Schlesinger 1996).

It is difficult to keep in mind the seeming paradox that change for the bet-ter can be bad for one's mental health. Treatment of severely traumatized patients is an arduous task, and it is a natural reaction on achieving signifi-cant improvement to enjoy it with a patient. Unexpected suicides at the mo-ment of special leaps forward in apparent recovery are tragic reminders of the complexities and dangers inherent in the treatment of traumatized pa-tients. Thus, the experience of severe trauma does not end with the cessation of violence. It continues to be reenacted in repetitive versions of the rela-tionship between victim and victimizer, and this relationship inevitably comes to dominate the transference at some point, taking many shapes and forms. Significant positive change signals to the patient the impending loss of the highly pathological but richly dramatic and complex transference with the therapist, and their trusting and supportive one as well. It is only when the fabric of envy, hatred, mutual seduction, and torture that constitutes the negative transference has been explored and resolved that change may become fully tolerable and stable.

CHAPTER 10

Erotic Transferences and Countertransferences

The psychotherapeutic situation is unlike any other two-person relationship: in everyday life, one does not experience the uninterrupted attentive listening of another person whose only intention is to be helpful. Patients who come to psychotherapy trustingly—with expectations, based on early comfortable and comforting experiences with benevolent adults, of being treated kindly—may respond to the unique psychotherapy situation with the so-called unobjectionable positive transference (Freud 1912) upon which a fruitful working alliance can be built. The therapist's attentive listening may stir feelings of appreciation and friendliness, and these may deepen into love with some sexual overtones.

To the extent that the treatment fosters or permits regression, such mild erotic transference may become a vehicle for archaic wishes; it constitutes a "resistance" in the sense that increasingly intense longings for the therapist's love preoccupy the patient and hinder the free expression of sexual and aggressive wishes that the patient fears would not be acceptable. It then becomes necessary to interpret the erotic transference as an obstacle to the goals of the treatment.

In the treatment of borderline patients, one rarely sees an initial, stable positive transference that gradually gives way to the erotic transference as resistance. Instead, these patients typically arrive at the first session with a welter of transferences that reflect their internal chaos. Their inner world is populated by "unmetabolized" self and object representations in intense aggressive and sexual relations with each other; they cannot but experience these various internalized object relationships, with aspects of themselves in interaction with imagined (projected) aspects of the therapist, and enact them in the sessions. Erotic preoccupation with the therapist may be for some of these patients a way to impose order and continuity on their inner turmoil; others focus on hostile, rejecting stances in the service of the same need.

EROTIC TRANSFERENCES AND
BOUNDARY VIOLATIONS IN THE
TREATMENT OF BORDERLINE PATIENTS

The reactions of therapists to patients' expressions of loving and sexual feelings toward them are perhaps the most common source of boundary violations in psychotherapy. This must come as no surprise, given that being loved and found attractive are experiences that people prize and enjoy in everyday life; the need to be desired and valued is universal and hence cannot be regarded as "pathological" in itself. Further, people commonly express and acknowledge loving or sexual feelings nonverbally by offering and accepting gifts, in subtle flirtatious gestures or direct sexual advances. Converting such communications into words often seems to deprive them of their emotional charge or to render them less pleasing or to expose the speaker to ridicule or rejection. If one fails to reciprocate another's expressions of affection, it shames him, and arousing shame is uncomfortable for the person who inflicts it. Indeed, for anyone who values human relationships, it is always painful to repel another's request for affection or tenderness. Hence, therapists in the presence of patients' seemingly "normal" expressions of affection often feel ill at ease. Sometimes they are aware of reciprocal feelings toward the patient and respond by becoming inhibited and behaving in an excessively formal manner so as to keep the patient at arm's length (Gabbard 1994).

Beyond these issues of courtesy and reticence is the fact that sexual feelings have in fact deep, momentous, and often terrifying aspects (Wrye and Welles 1989; Wrye 1993), for patients and therapists alike. On an unconscious level, sexual feelings are entangled with violent and shameful fantasies (Kernberg 1999) whose deepest origins in infancy are not accessible to semantic memory and hence are rarely reached in psychoanalytic treatment, let alone examined in ordinary introspection. For these and many other reasons, therapists are often tempted to avoid letting themselves be aware of their own or the patient's sexual and erotic feelings until their manifestations threaten to become unmanageable. The fear of primitive sexuality places the therapist at risk of acting on erotic feelings instead of privately examining his own feelings and helping the patient verbally express and examine hers.

CASE EXAMPLES

A beginning psychiatrist expressed doubts as to her fitness to practice psychotherapy because she had experienced sexual feelings toward some of her patients. She believed that "doctors shouldn't have those feelings toward patients." She was surprised and relieved to learn that all of a therapist's feelings can provide important information about the patient and the relationship being activated in the therapy, that it is as impossible to legislate one's own feelings as to forbid patients to feel one way or another, and that what matters is the therapist's ability to accept and examine feelings and put them into words rather than enacting them thoughtlessly or attempting to extinguish them.

The inability to tolerate or manage the conflation of sexuality with aggression accounts for much of the psychopathology of borderline patients. When these patients express erotic feelings in psychotherapy, it is almost always with a confusing admixture of hostility and coerciveness, which in turn evokes mixed feelings in the therapist. Lack of awareness of the full panoply of feelings evoked with special intensity by patients with severe personality disorders accounts in large measure for the tendency of therapists to cross boundaries when treating these patients. In an effort to manage their discomfort in the face of a patient's expressions of longing for love and sexual fulfillment, therapists can find themselves offering solace to soften the rejection that the patient fears and that the therapist feels in response to the aggressive component of the patient's message of longing and desperation.

Dr. G., a kindly and well-intentioned psychiatrist treating a lonely, penniless, and beautiful young woman, began to make house calls when she became ill with "chronic fatigue syndrome." He saw himself in the role of the famous Dr. Breuer, who, in collaboration with his patient "Anna O.," invented the "talking cure" that later became psychoanalysis. Unlike Breuer, however, who reacted to his patient's manifestations of love for him by taking flight, Dr. G. was unaware of being at risk of an unmanageable relationship. His compassion for his patient took the form of undertaking to support her when her funds were exhausted, and soon he found himself yielding to her pleas that he not leave her, as she could not live without him. By the time he sought consultation five years later, he and his patient were married and the parents of a baby; his wife remained suicidal, and Dr. G. was desperate.

The case of Dr. G. illustrates the concept of the "slippery slope" that can lead from simple acts of kindness to the inextricable and mutually disastrous involvement of unwitting therapists with ill, desperate, and appealing patients. In the decades since the unfortunate Dr. G. was lost to the field of psychiatry, therapists increasingly have found themselves in court or in trouble with their professional societies, accused of boundary violations. Many of these accusations (some valid, others imagined or trumped up) have been instigated by their borderline patients. Meanwhile, so much has been written about boundary violations in recent years, and so many caveats, laws, and rules have been raised to prevent them, that therapists' concerns about the consequences of crossing boundaries sometimes obliterate their ability to think psychologically about the manifestations of love, erotism, and sexuality that are an integral part of any psychotherapy (Gabbard and Lester 1995). To complicate the matter even further, the term "erotic transference" is often used loosely. Some clarification of this and related concepts may be in order.

THE CONCEPT OF EROTIC TRANSFERENCE

The *Concise Oxford Dictionary* definition of *erotic* suggests why there is lack of clarity about the term: *erotic* is defined as "of love, amatory," while *erotism* is defined as "sexual desire or excitement." Thus, love and sexual desire are conflated in the term, although, of course, they may occur independently.

The original term in English for the erotic transference was "transference love" (Freud 1915), a designation taken up by subsequent authors as if to imply that "transference" love was something special, distinct from "real" love. This implication suited the wish of both patients and therapists to distance themselves from their respective erotic responses to each other. Yet love is a natural response to the therapy situation, and the absence of such a response signals that something is missing, either in the patient's personality or in the treatment, because psychotherapy and psychoanalysis intrinsically promote the development of love for the therapist. People characteristically fall in love with someone who has power and authority in a situation favorable to regression—students fall in love with their teachers, hospital patients with their nurses, actors with their directors (Bergmann 1994). Love is more likely to flare up when the participants are together in privacy over a considerable length of time in situations that are relatively safe from the sobering implications of commitment (the shipboard or summer camp romance, or psychotherapy, with its at least initial assumption of an ending). The very conditions of emotional safety established explicitly by the treatment contract and implicitly (at first) in the minds of the patient and the therapist are conducive to falling in love. Martin Bergmann remarks: "It is a historical paradox that Freud, who found a way of cultivating a 'hothouse' variety of love, became concerned when analysands insisted on sexual gratification" (p. 509). That "transference love" is as real as any other form of love is now generally accepted; the term has been replaced by "erotic transference" to refer to a spectrum of behaviors activated in psychotherapies that foster or permit regression.

Therapists have sensed for years the distinction between an "erotic" transference, with its mixture of love and desire, and borderline patients' aggressively contaminated protestations. The distinction was finally conceptualized by Harold Blum (1973) in his influential paper in which he identified as an "erotized" transference "an intense, vivid, irrational erotic preoccupation with the analyst, characterized by overt, seemingly ego-syntonic demands for love and sexual fulfillment" (p. 63). He saw this as the extreme end of a spectrum of erotic transference manifestations, ranging from "productive positive transferences of affection and friendliness, through various subtle and not so subtle forms of seduction, to, finally, the extreme erotized form" (Hill 1994, p. 187).

It is a common experience for neurotic patients in psychotherapy or analysis to begin at the mildly affectionate, appreciative end of Blum's continuum, where they stir reciprocal feelings in the therapist, and to move through the middle reaches of the spectrum as regression occurs. At the end of successful transference analysis, grateful and affectionate feelings, perhaps mingled with sexual desire and mourning over its disappointment, may resurface. There are disagreements among therapists as to the accuracy of naming these end-phase feelings "transference," and the therapist's friendly, proud, benevolent, internal response "countertransference," when both parties are responding emotionally to a piece of work well done and to a relationship whose ending is bittersweet.

The erotized transference, most often encountered in treating borderline patients, derives its qualities of urgency, coerciveness, and irrationality from the fact that it uses the language of love and desire (both verbally and in actions) to express in disguise quite unloving wishes–to overpower, threaten, frighten, corrupt, humiliate, or disparage the therapist and to extort manifestations of love and desire. In so doing, patients seek to repair, through revenge, the wounds inflicted by traumatizing adults in their childhood or to confirm their belief that all persons in statu parentis are corrupt–or the whole world is. They may be trying to overcome deep feelings of helplessness, to shed feelings of shame or fear, by arousing them in the therapist, or to protect themselves from assault by becoming the attacker.

CASE EXAMPLE

Ms. L., an uncommonly beautiful young woman, endlessly repeated to her doctor her conviction that she was ugly, and that the only way he could persuade her that she was not as repulsive as she felt would be to make love to her. Indeed, on several occasions she began to disrobe or tried to fling herself into his arms.

Ms. N. campaigned at length for an affair with her doctor, pointing out that they both knew of analysts who had married their patients and angrily reproaching him for being unwilling to acknowledge sexual desire toward her and to marry her. She proclaimed herself to be more than willing to throw everything away–her treatment, her job, her little daughter (who could be sent off to live with her father)—out of passion for her doctor. That he was unwilling even to show her the warmth of an embrace proved that he was cold and unfeeling, that in fact he did not care for her at all and probably cared for no one but himself. His lack of reckless passion proved him, she maintained, to be a coward.

Mr. S. sent his therapist an elaborate bouquet on Valentine's Day to express his appreciation for her kindness and consideration.

These examples have in common their effect on the therapist, who, in each instance, felt vaguely coerced, uncomfortable, and helpless. Ms. L.'s therapist felt that her demand that he tell her she was beautiful indicated that if he did not do so she would conclude that he lacked a normal capacity to respond to her. He found himself half believing she was right. She further implied that his failure to love her would hurt her terribly and compel her to injure or kill herself. He felt terrorized and undermined rather than loved and desired. Similarly Ms. M.'s therapist felt confused and uneasy in the presence of his patient's "passion": perhaps, he thought, he was in fact somehow tepid and deficient by comparison with her abandon and intensity; perhaps he really was pathologically narcissistic. Mr. S.'s therapist felt that he was making a sexual advance toward her but did not want to hurt his feelings and was uncertain as to how to respond to his expensive gift. In each case, the patient expressed desires to control, coerce, and embarrass the therapist-as-transference-object nonverbally while cloaking those desires in erotic language and behavior. This made the patient's aggressive urge more difficult to identify as such. By listening to and understanding their own emotional responses, the therapists ultimately were able to deal effectively with their patients' confusing messages, accepting the normal components of longing and acknowledging and interpreting the rage and coercion.

In addition to the erotization of aggressive wishes and fantasies as a way of keeping them out of awareness, patients may also sexualize experiences not usually regarded as sexual as a way of expressing sexual wishes toward the therapist while not acknowledging them as such. Ms. M. presented a demure, dependent, deferential, "little girl" attitude toward her therapist, professing a maidenly horror of sex as dirty and shameful. At the same time, she gradually elaborated in the treatment a fantasy of cutting herself, bleeding almost to the point of death, being taken unconscious to the hospital, and awakening to find the concerned face of the therapist hovering over her. A second fantasy was of being tied to a hospital bed to prevent self-injury and waiting, in a state of rapturous anticipation, for her therapist to come and "assess" the risk of releasing her from restraints. She described both fantasies as "delicious." This patient disavowed sexual feelings toward the therapist and displaced them onto these fantasies, which gave expression not only to "delicious" masochistic sexual desires but also to her sadistic wishes to horrify and worry the therapist and to render him helpless.

EROTIC AND EROTIZED TRANSFERENCES
IN VARIOUS BORDERLINE SYNDROMES

Borderline pathology has the distinguishing hallmark of identity diffusion. That and the typical difficulty in dealing with aggression make the transference of genuinely erotic feelings unlikely to occur before successful integration of the fragmented, unconscious, internalized object relations that make up the inner world of these patients has been accomplished. Many therapists have noted with some bemusement their lack of sexual or affectionate responses to frankly sexual overtures or expressions of love from borderline patients—a reaction to the therapist's sense (perhaps unconscious) of the aggression disguised by the surface erotism.

Patients with narcissistic personality disorders rarely express loving feelings toward their therapists. These feelings activate the dependency wishes that such patients dread and cannot tolerate because of the envy and humiliation with which they are associated. Narcissistic patients' lack of apparent emotional investment in the therapist, then unconscious efforts to control him, and their devaluation of him as a defense against envy typically arouse intense insecurity in the therapist (Kernberg 1999).

Male patients with a narcissistic personality disorder, however, often sexualize the therapy situation with female therapists as a way to intimidate the therapist (Appelbaum and Diamond 1993). In these situations, the therapist must deal with considerable anxiety until she recognizes the patient's behavior as a means to prevent himself from experiencing feelings of dependency and as an outcome of the narcissist's inevitable envy of the therapist's capacity for genuine relationships.

In general, the shape and trajectory of the erotic transference and countertransference are determined by multiple factors that include the gender of each member of the therapy couple, the character traits and psychopathology of each, the prevailing, culturally sanctioned distributions of power and authority between men and women, and cultural attitudes toward sexuality and love (Kernberg 1999).

TECHNICAL ISSUES WITH EROTIC TRANSFERENCES IN BORDERLINE PATIENTS

The cornerstone of treatment of borderline patients is the treatment contract, which establishes from the outset that the relationship into which the patient and therapist are entering is not an ordinary one: rather, "whatever feelings are evoked in either one of them, be it love or aggression, will be examined and put in the service of the . . . therapy" (Bergmann 1999, p. 516). Bergmann's summary refers to an implicit aspect of the contract, namely, the expectation that the therapist will examine his feelings in private and then put the results of such self-reflection at the service of the treatment. Explicitly stated in the contract, aside from agreements about time and money, is the plan for managing the patient's behaviors that would be likely to interfere with the treatment. The work of establishing the contract clears the field for therapy in that when the patient breaks the contract (as inevitably occurs), the rupture can be interpreted in terms of the transference. Explicitly establishing the boundaries of the treatment helps to guarantee the physical and emotional safety of both participants, thus increasing the likelihood that the therapist will remain in his therapeutic role when the storms of the erotized transference make their appearance. It is in situations like the one precipitated by Ms. L. that the therapist may be most beleaguered; he will then be sustained by recognizing that at such moments it is necessary to abandon technical neutrality and take a stand on the side of the ego. Because the treatment is an enterprise of the ego, the therapist can unequivocally do whatever is necessary to preserve the treatment and afterward make clear to the patient why he thinks the patient had to provoke the crisis between them, and why he had to take protective action.

Hence, Ms. L.'s therapist first disentangled himself from her embrace, while telling her, "I don't like to reject or embarrass you, but I can't be a good therapist to you and let you behave this way." He then matter-of-factly requested that she put her shirt back on, and (upon catching his breath) went on to say, "In this work we are trying to do together, everything depends on our willingness to put feelings into words rather than acting on them. That's why I had to stop you. It's important to recognize that your threat to hurt or kill yourself if I refused to make love with you shows how intensely you need to feel that you can force me to act in accordance with your wishes, and that we are right now in a power struggle instead of a loving relationship." In subsequent sessions, the patient and therapist began to understand some of the fear behind her coercive behavior, including its origin in childhood trauma. (As discussed in chapter 9, evidence is building in the literature for trauma as a major instigator of borderline pathology in general; it also leads to a propensity to develop an erotized transference; cf. Bergmann 1999, p. 15.)

In his calm management of Ms. L.'s attempt at seduction and his prompt reinstatement of technical neutrality in the subsequent interpretation of what had happened, Ms. L.'s therapist avoided some common errors in dealing with patients' expressions of erotic or erotized feelings. One of these is the misuse of interpretation in the service of moving the erotic mo-ment out of the relationship with the therapist and into the past: "It is not now, it was then"; "it is not with me, it is with your parents." Thus, an "in-terpretation" such as, "What you feel for me is really a repetition of what you felt for your father as a little girl," is in fact a full retreat from the anx-ious moment of feeling the patient's urgency and the therapist's own fear: the therapist disavows his own, personal implication in the erotized scene by invoking the parents of the patient's childhood; he retreats from the here and now to the past; and he retreats from the reality of the patient's feelings ("What you *really* feel . . . ") to an implied disparagement of the patient's feelings as "mere" transference.

A second defense that therapists (especially beginners) raise against their own erotic feelings and those of the patient is to invoke external authority: "It is against the rules of the clinic for me to give you the hug you are asking for." Here the effort is to close the subject while dodging the patient's angry reaction. "I would gladly give you a hug were it not for the rules, so don't blame me for refusing you." The implicit seductiveness of this response can only fuel a patient's fantasy that the therapist would be available were she to end the treatment and free both of them from "the rules of the clinic."

False reassurance is still another means of deflecting rather than acknowl-edging and interpreting the reality of the patient's feelings. In response to the urgent request of the patient that he tell her "how you really feel about me–you hate me, I know," the therapist responds, "No, of course I don't hate you, I feel warmly toward you. But our job here is to try to understand your feelings, not mine." Here the therapist unconsciously (or perhaps not so un-consciously) hopes that by tossing the patient a crumb (warm feelings), he can hold at bay her peremptory need for full affirmation of her desirability. His denial of hating her sidesteps the issue of her projected hateful feelings. On the surface, he is implicitly representing himself as devoid of the angry and retaliatory feelings that the patient unconsciously knows she has every reason to expect him to have in response to her coercive behavior. His stiff reminder of what their "job" is represents his loss of neutrality as he takes on the role of father or schoolmaster sternly bringing her back into line. Her response is either to feel properly chastised and to try not to evoke his stern-ness again, or to be enraged by the disingenuousness of his statement.

Focusing on the aggressive elements in the erotization of the transference without giving equal recognition to the sensitive issues of longing, embarrassment, desire, and shame can rob treatment of the erotized transference of half its potential as a means of arriving at deeper understanding. Therapists typically find it easier to deal with aggression and violence than with their patients' erotic feelings and wishes. Thus, when an erotic transference is unverbalized, the therapist may be content to let well enough alone. The result can be either escalation to unmanageable enactments or a vitiated treatment terminated prematurely. A therapist who is as alert to signs of love as to those of hate can acknowledge the reality of such feelings and tactfully find a way for them to be expressed and understood.

In summary, therapists commonly experience patients' persistent importunings for love and sexual fulfillment as an even greater strain on their composure than the experience of being attacked, reviled, and ridiculed. In staving off another's offer of love or refusing a request for it, one risks humiliating the other; to a person in the grip of desire, any response other than acceptance or reciprocation feels like a rejection. But just as resistance was seen at first as an obstacle to analysis and later came to be appreciated as an opportunity to approach more closely the truth of inner experience, and as countertransference was originally a source of analysts' private shame and later became a source of enlightenment about the patient-therapist relationship (largely owing to the work of Heinrich Racker [1968]), so a patient's expressions of love, longing, and desire and the therapist's reflection on his own responses can inform and advance the treatment.

The therapist who can use the patient's erotic transference to the advantage of the treatment has to be sturdy, steady, and open-minded, assiduously seeking an honest, mutually accepting relationship with the patient. To this end, he provides a safe setting in which neither the patient nor the therapist is endangered, thus enabling the inner life of the patient to be revealed and expressed as transference rather than as somatic illness or destructive action. This therapist tolerates long periods of being alternately importuned and attacked without retaliating or withdrawing, instead remaining capable of empathizing both with the patient's enjoyment of being abusive or seductive and with the fears that lie beneath these behaviors. Meanwhile, the therapist continues to try to help the patient become aware of the hatred and envy that are disguised by aggressive erotic advances and to acknowledge how humiliated, pained, guilty, and scared it makes the patient to experience and express these feelings. The therapist remains alert to the likelihood that attacks on the "bad," withholding therapist reflect the hope that the "good," trustworthy one will eventually emerge. This is "emotional holding and cognitive containing." It can lead to the elucidation of the wish that the therapist heal the wounds of childhood and to the patient's discovery of some of the infantile sources of the search for pleasure and affection in adult life.

PART THREE
DRAWING ON COMPLEMENTARY RESOURCES

CHAPTER 11

Using Dream Material

In his famous monograph of 1899, Freud spoke of dreams as the royal road to the unconscious. Dream analysis became an important element, often the mainstay, in the psychoanalytic treatment of neurotic patients. In psychodynamic psychotherapies of borderline patients, such as TFP, dreams may emerge quite prominently and dramatically. Often these dreams present stark and quite primitive imagery that, as we discuss later in this chapter, may provide indications of the patient's ego strength and level of personality organization. In addition, dreams appearing in the treatment of borderline patients may provide important information about central dynamic issues, the meaning of the transference, and the significance of acting out. This channel of information may be particularly valuable in treating those borderline patients who are extremely inhibited in what they can discuss with the therapist, as well as those in whom splitting keeps crucial information out of the sessions.

DREAM ANALYSIS IN THE
THERAPY OF BORDERLINE PATIENTS

Borderline patients, whether diagnosed according to the criteria of *DSM-IV* or to the broader criteria (emphasizing personality organization) of Otto Kernberg (1967), are often more secretive and less forthcoming about their inner life than is routinely the situation with better integrated ("neurotic") patients. Sometimes this lack of candor constitutes a major stumbling block to the therapeutic work, since the therapist may come to feel quite puzzled and in the dark as to what is going on with the patient at any given moment. This is particularly worrisome when the therapist has reason to suspect that the patient is acting out—in the literal sense of en-acting certain key feelings in the transference through inappropriate and impulsive behaviors in the outside world. Moreover, these behaviors may have a decidedly self-destructive edge to them: they may not only keep crucial verbal material unavailable for the therapeutic encounter but actu-ally threaten the welfare of the patient. This is not, of course, to say that neurotic patients in classical psychoanalytic treatment are immune to the phenomenon of resistance—keeping material hidden from the analyst, ei-ther through repression, where the material is unconscious, or through withholding, where the patient is fully aware. On the contrary, resistance is a universal phenomenon in analytic therapy, or indeed, in any form of extended therapy. But neurotic patients are less prone to acting out and seldom place themselves in the life-threatening situations that are the hall-mark of the borderline patient.

CASE EXAMPLE

In the following example, a borderline patient's serious acting out was at first not easily linked with the transference situation. The connection even-tually became clear through the "intermediary" of a dream reported while the acting-out behaviors were taking place.

A woman of twenty-two was being treated at a psychiatric hospital, where she had been admitted some months before because of suicide ges-tures while at college. For several weeks, while out on weekend passes, she had begun to frequent bars in questionable areas of town. Her attractiveness guaranteed that she would win the notice of the men at these establish-ments. Selecting a man with tattoos and bulging muscles, she would go to his apartment, have sex, but then, as often as not, get beaten up by the man after provoking an argument or refusing to make another "date." Usually the men she ended up with were considerably older than herself. This string of events was happening shortly before the marriage of her therapist, which was common talk among the staff and patients of her unit, but about which she professed to have no reaction whatsoever.

She reported having the following two dreams on the same night:

I am encased in a plastic bubble. There are people milling about on the outside, at a party apparently, having a good time. I push at the walls of the bubble, but it won't give, so I'm stuck inside.

I'm walking along a street in a deserted part of town. All of a sudden, there are some green monsters in back of me, running and trying to catch me. I run as fast as I can, but they're gaining on me. I wake up just before they are about to grab me.

Her associations to the first dream led her to thoughts about her mounting sense of isolation, of being cut off from the world of people who were having fun and enjoying themselves. The second dream remained elusive for her until she was asked to focus on the color of the monsters: What did green call to mind? She recalled that people sometimes referred to envy in that way: there was the expression "green with envy." Reluctantly, she then began to talk about the therapist's upcoming marriage, which not only meant a separation of two weeks because of the honeymoon but also a change in his life, signifying that he now had a life partner and a sexual partner while she continued to languish in the hospital, sans friend, sans mate, sans lover. She could begin to see that her impulsive seeking of sexual partners was driven by a desire not only to emulate her therapist but to have *him* as her partner. A proud woman from a socially prominent family, it was embarrassing and uncomfortable for her to admit that she could care that much about someone as "ordinary" as her therapist in the first place. She eventually understood that a punishment for sexual pleasure was built into her choice of sexual partners—rough men in their thirties or forties who mistreated her. It was the price she had to pay, in effect, for what amounted to "illicit" sex with father-substitutes (who were, to this extent, stand-ins for the therapist as well).

*   *   *

The way in which dreams can point to otherwise hidden dynamics in a borderline patient, and even provide indications of the patient's future behavior, was highlighted in the following case. A high school student of seventeen was referred for therapy after her release from a hospital where she had been admitted because of a suicide gesture. She and her older sister lived with their father, a corporate executive. The father had a "Jekyll and Hyde" personality: he was jovial and polite with everyone else, but physically and verbally abusive, ill tempered, and hypercritical with his daughters. He was apparently the same with their mother. The parents had argued constantly, and by the time the patient was five or six, the mother had effectively abandoned the family, taking up with a lover and spending only a minimal amount of time with the children. Around the time of the patient's eighth birthday, her mother was riding in a car driven by her lover when there was a collision with another car; the mother was hurled into the air and killed instantly.

The most striking aspect of the initial sessions with the girl was that she made no mention of her mother. Indirect allusions to her sense of abandonment, however, came through in her first dream:

> I was part of a family. I had a little sister. We were very poor. We wanted to have a nice Christmas, but we didn't have enough money to buy a tree. So we went to the forest to cut down a tree. My parents left me and my sister alone, so I tried to protect her. We were sad, but I didn't feel desperate because I was glad I was there for her; I had someone I loved.

Curiously, she was the younger sister, by four years, and her older sister helped to raise her, acting as a second mother. The maternal grandmother also helped fill this surrogate role. In the dream, the patient appeared to compensate for the disappearance of the mother by adopting the maternal role toward her "younger" sister: she "became" her mother by way of denying the loss. Her father had seemingly conspired to frustrate the acknowledgment of her mother's death—hampering the business of mourning—by refusing to let her go to her mother's funeral.

Ten days later, she reported the following dream:

> I am pregnant and in a hospital. The doctors and nurses take me by force, put me in a bed, and take away my baby. I fall asleep, and when I awaken, my father and sister are there, looking very mean at me. I run out and grab my son. I am happy and feel love for him. My father is furious with me. People take me up into a wooden house in the air, perched over a river where there are crocodiles. There are other girls with babies in that house. The hospital people and my father want us to jump. I say I'm not going to jump. I am very frightened, thinking they are going to push me so I will fall into the river.

The day residue had included the newspaper story about the U.S. marine plane that flew too low and severed a ski-cable in Italy, causing some twenty skiers to plunge to their death on the rocks below. This story was transformed into a scenario in which she now had a baby of her own—someone to love and be loved by, someone who could never be taken from her. Only it was taken from her by the cruel father and hospital personnel. They even ordered her to commit suicide.

At the time of this dream, she did not have a boyfriend, much less any immediate plans to get pregnant. Because of her father's abusiveness, she had taken to living with friends, spending almost no time at home. She had little motivation for treatment and often skipped appointments. Interpretations to the effect that she seemed, below the surface, preoccupied with the theme of motherhood, her dead mother, and her wishes to make up for the grievous loss of her mother by becoming one herself—all fell on deaf ears.

Related themes cropped up, nevertheless, in her dreams from a month later:

I am with my father high up on our balcony. My cat jumps off the balcony. My father says, "Don't worry about it—it'll land on its feet." I'm afraid it'll die or get lost in the city. A woman from the ground floor of the building says, "Oh, your cat's fine: it's with me."

This was followed by a dream in which

I'm with some kids in the village in Italy where I grew up. One of the guys gets aggressive with me and says we have to get married! I feel I have to go along with it because he has power over me. I then see his father talking to my father. My father is looking very mean.

The cat falling off the balcony was an allusion to the traumatic death of her mother; her attachment to her cat was intense, and she herself could acknowledge that the love she felt for it was like a substitute for the closeness she had wanted, but never had, with her mother. This was as close as she came to her emotions about the as-yet unmourned mother. Why did the boy say she had to marry him? She said that he was probably insisting that she marry him because he had gotten her pregnant, though there was no particular boy she had in mind and she had not been conscious lately of wanting a baby.

A few weeks later, the patient left treatment, ostensibly to have more time to study for her spring exams. Nearer to the truth, as the therapist saw it, was her disinclination to get any closer to the painful emotions surrounding the loss of her mother—all the more painful because of the decade-long abusiveness from her father that began within days, as she recalled, after her mother's death.

At all events, two years after she left treatment, her older sister sought treatment with the same therapist, her problem being one of depression with feelings of worthlessness and occasional thoughts of suicide (never acted out). She reported that her sister had returned to Europe after finishing high school in the United States, that she had quickly become infatuated with a young man she met in her native town—and that she was now three months pregnant by him. She was determined to have the baby—who would be born out of wedlock, just as the older sister was. (Their parents had married sometime between the births of the two girls.) The younger sister's life course, in other words, was following the "script" laid out in her earlier pregnancy dream—about which the older sister, of course, knew nothing. In keeping with her tendency to act out her feelings connected with the mother's death rather than to work them out verbally in therapy, the younger sister had gone ahead and become pregnant, swearing her sister to secrecy (lest their father get enraged and try to thwart her will) and revealing the news only after the pregnancy had progressed past the time when abortion would still have been possible.

*   *   *

The older sister, although she also functioned at a borderline level, was better integrated. The younger sister, for example, met *DSM-IV* criteria for borderline personality disorder, whereas the older sister, who did not meet these criteria, showed a dysthymic picture and a depressive-masochistic character structure. Her dreams did not contain images of mutilation or dying but did have a primitive quality of a kind often noted in borderline patients. In her first dream, for example, she envisioned that

> little spiders are crawling on me as I'm in bed. Baby spiders. There is a big spider on the wall that is about to explode and more little spiders would burst forth. If I pour honey on the big spider, I figure I can placate it.

A patient's first dream while in therapy is said to encapsulate her main dynamic(s)—her whole "neurosis" in a nutshell, as it were. The older sister's associations led in several interrelated directions. When her sister was little, a spider laid eggs in her skin, causing a kind of pimple. The patient had gone the day before to the Museum of Modern Art, where she saw a painting of insects. The big spider was pumping like a heart. The year before, she had become pregnant by her boyfriend and had had an abortion. She was very scared of spiders. This put her in mind of her father, of whom she was also very scared because of his irascibility.

Several days later, she reported two brief dreams. In the first:

I am in bed, and I want to have sex with my father.

This was immediately followed by:

My feelings change, and I don't want to have sex with my father, only he forces himself on me.

In reality, she does not believe that her father molested her sexually. He did seem conflicted about her, in the sense that he would leer at her in a sexual way at times or behave immodestly around the house, as though he found her quite attractive. Outwardly, however, he could be counted on to be critical, even mocking of her, upbraiding her, for instance, for "smelling bad" even after she came out of the bath, or for having a "disgusting hairdo" right after she came from the beauty parlor. She began to feel that he had actually been struggling to contain his sexual feelings toward her—by depreciating her vociferously and by denying his attraction altogether. She could also begin to acknowledge that she was torn in a similar way, disliking him to the point of near-hatred, yet experiencing at times an attraction to him as a successful, socially polished, and good-looking man. When she and her sister were in their early teens, their father remarried; their stepmother subsequently told the older sister once that the father had done something sexual with the younger girl. Whether this was true is unclear. What seemed more clear was that, as the dream material and her associations suggested, a love-hate relationship existed between the father and both girls, with strong (though suppressed) sexual undercurrents on either side. This came through in the orgastic quality of the spider dream—the big spider exploding with all the little spiders—which she had at a time when she was beginning to glimpse the hidden side of the father-daughter relationship. Bringing this material to the surface in the therapy had a beneficial, not to say liberating, effect: she no longer saw herself as a disgusting and worthless person, a pariah whom no one would want to be around. She could begin to understand that her father may well have needed to cast her (and her younger sister) in such an unfavorable light as a defense against the incestuous impulses with which he seemed for so many years to have been struggling.

*   *   *

The next example illustrates how work with dreams can facilitate the emergence of important sexual issues in a borderline patient with problems in the area of sexual identity. This patient's sense of what was "proper" to talk about helped her to rationalize her strong denial defenses and led to an evasiveness in sessions.

A woman in her late forties had been hospitalized briefly following a suicide gesture. This had been precipitated by a sexual affair with a woman from her bridge club, the first experience she had had with a same-sex love affair. She was married with three children. Her husband, a successful businessman, had been attractive to her originally as a strong, protective figure. Earlier in her life, she had been sexually molested by her grandfather (though without intercourse). Reared in a very form-conscious family in which one had to maintain the appearance that everything was "fine," she did not feel free to reveal the incestuous experiences to her family; when she finally did so years later, she was rebuffed by her mother, who waved the matter aside, saying, "That happens to all of us; just forget it and get on with your life." She was more fond of her father, though he was an alcoholic and, when drinking, was irritable and violent. His many affairs with young women eventually became known and led to divorce. The patient continued to "maintain appearances" throughout her married life but harbored deep-seated distrust and dislike of men. These feelings she was able to suppress until her children were nearly grown, at which point a largely intolerable situation loomed: life reduced to just herself and her husband. Her husband continued to be very protective of her, but she felt little closeness to him because of his quite different values and interests. It was in this setting that she tumbled, to her own bewilderment, into the affair with a woman acquaintance.

Over the course of her therapy, which consisted of analytically oriented sessions three times a week, her dreams made clear the underlying dynamics in a way that would have been difficult to unearth otherwise, given her reticence about sexual matters in general and her strong need to maintain a facade of "normalcy."

The following was the first dream she reported in treatment:

There is an animal's head on a table, connected to its body, which is under the table. Someone tries to lift the head off the table, and I shout, "No! You'll hurt the animal!" But the person doesn't listen to me and lifts the head right off the animal, which is torn apart in the process and killed.

The allusions here were, on the surface, to her husband's tendency, as she experienced it, to "not listen to her." The danger in this inattention was serious: the death of the "animal" (herself). The man seen as handling the creature very roughly was reminiscent of her grandfather and her often irascible and out-of-control father.

A week later, she had another dream:

I walk out of a building with some girls. We see a big snake coiled up. I warn them: "It could strike out at a distance of five feet!" I was afraid the girls would get hurt or poisoned.

This was the first of many "snake" dreams. Her associations at this point centered on the danger she connected with men and on what they can inflict on women. The "danger" is general for her, not specifically sexual.

Two weeks later:

I'm in a car with one of my daughters, going over a dirt road. We go off the main road over some rough terrain. There is a pile of boulders beyond which we can't go. In the distance, we see a crashed airplane, and a person crushed in the wreckage.

The main road she equated with heterosexuality; going off it represented homosexuality. The crushed person was herself—caught and overwhelmed in the no longer satisfying marital situation but frightened at the implications of having been ensconced in a homosexual relationship.

Two months later:

I walk into the kitchen with my mother and one of my daughters. There're two huge spiders near a huge web. I tell them to walk away. One of the spiders is close to mother. The spider drops onto me. I cry out, "They're on me!'"

She spoke of feeling suffocated when her husband tried to be affectionate, as when he put his arm around her. It was "creepy" when her uncle used to touch her all over. I wondered whether the "spider close to her mother" was her father—who was a frightening man in his own way. She made no reference to him in this session.

A week later:

> As I back out of the garage, I see the shadow of a man wearing a hat. The "shadow" comes closer, walking toward my side of the car. I cry out, "No, oh no!"

It wasn't clear who the "old man" was: she spoke more of her grandfather, who first began to "grope" her right in front of his wife. The fear of men, at all events, had spread to her husband, who never forced himself on her and was not a womanizer and alcoholic like her father. The dream had a nightmare quality and made the therapist think of past experiences with men that had been distinctly traumatic for her, though thus far the therapist knew only about the grandfather.

Two weeks later:

> I watch a man put his hand and arm in the ground right through the dirt. As he withdraws it, it is all bloody. There are guts hanging out of his hand—that seem to belong to the body of a woman he'd killed: the body was decomposing.

The dream had a primitive quality, like the dreams occasionally seen in borderline and psychotic persons that feature mutilated bodies and blood and gore. She spoke of feeling "dead" the past two years, as a result of having been "killed," spiritually, by what men had done to her. Her extreme anger at her grandfather and her fear of her father had been displaced of late onto her husband. Some of these feelings were meant for the therapist, she began to recognize, if only because he urged her to bring these issues to the surface and to deal with them, whereas she would have preferred to sweep all this painful material under the rug.

A month later:

> I look for the bathroom in our old house. I turn and see my father, and I say hello. His eyes are all black. He hugs me and says, "I love you, honey."

The bathroom imagery comes up again and again in her dreams. Something important must have happened there. But what? And something is putting the spotlight on her ambivalent relationship with her father: a lovable monster.

A week later:

> I'm in a bathroom with a small window behind a toilet. As I start to walk out, I
> see that someone has broken through the window and come through. I cry out,
> "Mommy!"

She likened the glass shattering to the threatened breakup of her family. The dream also carried an allusion to the past: something about a frightening experience in a bathroom, and the presence in it of another person (her father?).

A few days later:

> I hide from a man who is searching for me. I get into bed with a woman and get
> close to her under the covers, so that it'll look like we are just one person. The
> scene changes, and I hear someone crashing through a window.

She could begin to see that the threat to her safety came from men: her grandfather, her father. Security lay in closeness to her mother—who in real life failed to protect her from the dangers stemming from men. But she sought this refuge in the homosexual relationship, where she could not only feel safe but have a comforting sense of "oneness" with her lover. She recalled that, when she was eleven, her father got angry at her mother because her mother had danced with her brother in law. The father, drunk, had kicked in the front door of the house. The patient had cleaned him up in the bathroom—perched him on the toilet and cleaned him up.

A week later:

> I go to the bathroom in our old house—the one I grew up in. The door slowly
> opens. A hand comes around the door. I cry out: "Oh no!" and then I cry,
> "Daddy!"

The sense of being cornered reminded her of being cornered both by her grandfather and by another more distant relative who also forced sex on her.

It was unclear to her in the dream whether her father was a potential rescuer from these men or simply another man who also frightened her and may have done something inappropriate.

Three weeks later, she reported a nightmare:

> I'm on my back. Opposite where I sleep is a bathroom. From out the bathroom door a figure emerges covered in black . . . even the face is covered. I feel frightened. I lift up the cover and scream, and I woke up.

She had only vague associations to the dark figure: it seemed to be a man, but she could not say who she thought it might be. The day residue included an approach by her husband, who had put his arm around her affectionately; irritated, she had been repulsed. But his actions fell short of the terror-inspiring circumstances of the dream, which pointed to her childhood experiences with men—probably her father in this case, since the dream was situated in her own childhood house.

A week later:

> I'm in a house. As I walk outside, there is a tarantula nearby. There are more of them under the foundations of the house. I step over them and warn some women in the house and tell them to call the exterminators.

She recalled her mother telling her that, when she used to work in the garden with her father, he would sometimes get very angry and she would run into the house crying. Her equation of spiders with scary men becomes clearer now. It seems that her grandfather and her father frightened her in different ways: her grandfather because of the sexual molestation; her father because of his anger and unpredictable, disturbing behavior when drunk. Whether there was also a sexual component to his frightening behavior seemed at first a possibility, but no compelling evidence had ever surfaced.

With this borderline patient, the dream sequences helped unearth the central dynamics, enabling us to get around her evasiveness about the past and around the defenses of denial, disavowal, and repression. Now that her children were about to leave home for college or work, she could look forward only to life with her husband. For her, this was too reminiscent of the early experiences with her father and grandfather. Expecting the "worst," and longing for closeness with a mothering figure—an element sorely lacking in her past—she escaped into a sexual relationship with a woman. She also sought a kind of protection from men, which her actual mother did not provide, but which a fantasied mother—in the person of the female lover—might offer her. This came at a price, however: loss of her husband and children, or at least of their support and affection. Her sense of entrapment stemmed from this conflict and had led to the suicide gesture, since at the time she saw no way out.

*   *   *

The following case illustrates how dreams highlighted the transference in a schizotypal borderline man. There are many roads that lead to transference interpretation: the patient's conversation when it focuses on intense feelings about "someone else," which serves as a thin screen for reference to the therapist; direct allusions to the therapist; dreams in which the symbolism seems clearly related to feelings about the therapist; and dreams in which the therapist is pictured literally and forcibly. The last type of dream occurs with some regularity in patients with fragile ego structure (borderline or psychotic). The following sequence of highly disturbing and blatantly transference-related dreams came from a schizotypal borderline man. He had been tormented during his childhood by a hypercritical, at times outright abusive, mother. This experience, interacting with his vulnerable constitution, had created in him a personality characterized by depressive and schizoid traits, self-injurious behavior, and extreme sensitivity to adverse comment. A highly intelligent and effective engineer, he fortunately met with little such criticism in his adult life, but what little came his way he experienced as devastating.

The following was his first dream while in treatment:

You [the therapist] are in my bed—dead. I wonder: *What am I going to do now?!* I figure I'll just keep you around. . . . Then I'll feel safe.

It is most unusual for a neurotic-level patient to incorporate the therapist in so undisguised a manner—and within the first few days of treatment. The therapist's appearance so early, especially as a kind of corpse-totem—eternally "there" (albeit dead) to ward off feelings of loneliness and unprotectedness—was in and of itself a signal to the fragile ego in this patient.

A week later:

You are a surgeon, and I am on the operating table. I am covered with glass, and you go, "Bang!" on my glass surface, and I fragment.

This dream signals vividly how terrified the patient was of his new therapist. He saw him as a doctor whose remarks could smash him into a thousand pieces. He also expressed the fear that the therapist might somehow "steal" his personality, adding: "I don't have much of a personality, so I'd be afraid of losing even that little bit." In reaction to stress, ever since childhood, he tended to dissociate, sometimes to the point of experiencing several "alters"—all with the same name, however. Some were "benign" and helpful; others were frightening.

Three weeks later:

You shot three of my other "selves."

He mentioned that during the therapist's weeklong absence he had had another dream in which the therapist appeared as a whale that swallowed him up. From a transference standpoint, this was a parallel to his early experiences with his mother, whose domineering personality had threatened to engulf him and to obliterate his burgeoning personality. Therapy remained a threatening process with life-or-death implications. Shooting some of his other "selves" had both good and bad aspects: it eliminated his false selves, making his real self preeminent, but at the high cost of destroying the "selves" on whom he had long relied for a sense of protection and for a surcease from loneliness.

A month later:

My father and I kill my mother and stuff her in a coffin.

In his everyday life, he had gotten on better with his parents in recent years, yet he still reacted to the world in ways reminiscent of his early years, when he could scarcely picture surviving unless his mother (and at times his father as well) were dead. Here again, the starkly undisguised nature of the dream is suggestive of ego fragility.

A few days later:

You and I are in a boxing match. I am angry with you.

He mentioned that these dreams and his tendency to dissociate were like what people who have been sexually abused may experience, yet he recalled no such events in his early years. He was still upset with the therapist for finding out about the other "selves," as though this would strip away his defenses before healthier ones could develop and take their place. Subsequent dreams, however, became more benign; the other "selves" receded into the background, seldom reappearing, and his mood brightened. The treatment had succeeded by this time in allaying some of his original anxieties; a more trusting alliance had begun to form.

DREAMS AS A
BAROMETER OF EGO STRENGTH

In the early psychoanalytic literature, little attention was paid to possible correlations between the manifest imagery of the dream and the diagnostic condition pertinent to the dreamer. That is, distinctions were not drawn between the manifest content of the dreams of higher-functioning neurotic patients versus those of more disturbed patients who were functioning at levels we would now designate as "borderline" or psychotic (Kernberg 1967).

In contradistinction to Freud's (1923) contention that the ego cannot conceive of its own death,[1] evidence (Stone 1979) shows that dreams of one's own death or severe mutilation can indeed occur, but that they are peculiar to patients who have poorly integrated personalities and who function at subneurotic levels, either borderline or psychotic.

Dreams of this type serve as neurophysiological "markers," betokening fragile ego structure. Accurately assessed, such dreams may also serve as a tip-off that the patient is more fragile than originally diagnosed. This could alert the therapist to the potential for paranoid regressions during the therapy (see chapter 7) and could also bring the therapist to consider the possibility of a misdiagnosis of a psychotic patient as borderline (see chapter 3).

---

[1] That is, one did not find dreams in which the dreamer pictured himself as literally dead—as opposed to dreams in which the dreamer's death will be an inevitable consequence of, say, falling off a cliff, except that the dreamer awakens before the curtain falls, so to say, on the last act.

CASE EXAMPLES OF MUTILATION DREAMS
AND DREAMS OF PRIMITIVE STARKNESS

A married woman of twenty-seven sought treatment because of a deteriorating marital situation. Her husband had become uncommunicative, speaking almost not a single word to her for several months. She had become depressed, lonely, and irritable, though she was continuing to work. She had never been in psychotherapy before, although both her sisters had been hospitalized because of suicide gestures and were considered borderline. A grandfather had been diagnosed as paranoid and bipolar manic-depressive.

During the second week of therapy, she reported the following dream:

> I am in a recovery room of a hospital. Arrayed all around me, on either side of
> my body, are the organs from my chest and abdomen: my kidneys, spleen,
> heart, liver. . . . My surgeon says hello but is quite drunk and slurs his speech as
> he tries to reassure me: "Thass okay, young lady, donchu' worry, ev'thin's
> gonna' be awright."

So extensive was the mutilation in this dream that by rights she should have been dead. The primitive and grotesque quality of the dream signified that her ego strength might be much more fragile than originally assumed. Her subsequent course was that of borderline personality disorder with impulsive suicidal acts, substance abuse, and stormy relationships. The content of the dream also pointed to important dynamics: her father, who died during her adolescence, had been a surgeon who abused alcohol. The transference implications were clear: she feared putting herself—and her life—in the hands of a new doctor, whom she could not trust at this early juncture any better than she could trust her tipsy surgeon-father.

*   *   *

A man of thirty-one had been married for nine years when his wife began to put pressure on him to get a mortgage and move, finally, to a real house. Older than her husband, she heard the tick of her "biological clock" and was eager to settle down and have a child. Her husband was psychologically unprepared for such a move but went along with her request. The day before the closing on the mortgage, he became acutely anxious and had the following dream:

I look down at my groin and see only a bloody stump where my penis should have been. My penis was lying on the ground, and blood was pouring out of my groin.

This man was hospitalized a few days later with an agitated depression and was also diagnosed with borderline personality disorder.

*   *   *

A young man with paranoid schizophrenia reported this dream:

I open the refrigerator, and I see two glasses of water. One of my eyeballs is in each glass, staring at me.

The dream is one of mutilation of the body: the eyes are separated from the rest of the person and, in a manner characteristic of paranoid persons (with their suspiciousness and hypervigilance), are staring at the patient. In this sense, the dream is reminiscent of findings in a study of schizophrenics' dreams (Richardson and Moore 1963): the qualities of bizarreness, mutilation of self and others, and blatant aggressivity toward others are present significantly more often than in nonschizophrenics ("The whole world is flushing its toilets, and the outlet is down my throat").

*   *   *

A twenty-eight-year-old homosexual man from the South had been diagnosed with borderline personality disorder. He went into a severe panic state after he asked his therapist to perform fellatio on him. The therapist refused and tried to explore the reasons why this wish surfaced at this particular time. The next night, the patient reported later, he had the following dream while still in a state of intense anxiety:

My father and I are in a plane flying over my mother, who is encased in concrete, in the lithotomy position, being fucked by a big black man. My father and I are dropping bombs of shit onto my mother from the plane.

Here the dream is striking not because of extensive mutilation (of a sort that would be fatal under ordinary circumstances) but because of its grotesque and undisguised aggressivity.

CASE EXAMPLES OF DREAMS
OF NEARLY DYING

Often during a time of crisis, the borderline patient reports to the therapist a dream in which he envisioned himself as almost dead—as in the process of dying but not quite dead. Insofar as this kind of dream may also occur in neurotic-level patients (especially at times of interpersonal crisis or after serious life events like a job loss), it is not an unequivocal index of more fragile (that is, borderline or psychotic) mental organization.

A borderline patient with schizotypal features reported the following dream:

> I was walking down a street in Nevada . . . very unfamiliar area. I could hardly breathe, it was so hot. Evil seemed to be all around me. I felt myself about to strangle. I could see indentations in my throat, as if someone's hands were around my neck. I was dying and was very scared. I felt a terrible pressure on my genitals and pelvic area, as though that whole area were about to be crushed.

This patient's therapist had just announced his summer vacation. The dream had the quality of a nightmare, from which the patient awoke uncomfortably. Dynamically, the dream alluded to homosexual feelings, which were mobilized by the patient's reaction to the temporary loss of his therapist. Projected onto the therapist, these feelings were seen as "crushing" the patient's genitals, loss and castration being equated in the process.

*   *   *

A married woman of twenty-eight, borderline with hysteric features, had the following dream at a time when her marriage was disintegrating and she was realizing that divorce was inevitable:

> I try to swim across a narrow river. But before I get to the other side, a shark bites off my leg, and I am stranded and bleeding to death in the middle of the water. I'm just about to pass out . . . when I awaken.

*   *   *

The following dream was reported by an obsessional man functioning at the neurotic level. His previous session had been canceled because the therapist had suddenly been called away for an emergency:

> I am in my laboratory. A man comes by, having stolen something. I accost him about being a thief. We are standing two feet apart. Suddenly I become aware that he has just stabbed me in the heart. I feel I am dying, and I start to cry out for help, but I am unable to. I fall in a heap. I pull out a dagger and stab him in the arm—not a fatal blow. I feel I can maybe hold out for another few minutes.

Here the "assailant" is the therapist, who has "robbed" him of a session. From an ego-psychological standpoint, the dream, in its manifest content, is not a total "failure" (as it would be if the dreamer saw himself as actually dead). The dreamer is not quite dead, as the dream ends, and he does get to strike a blow at the assailant, albeit an ineffective one.

CASE EXAMPLES OF DREAMS OF BEING DEAD

Dreams of being dead are predominantly reported by borderline patients. One such patient, a woman of twenty-two, had experienced incest at the hands of her father for several years between the ages of eight and thirteen. She reported the following dream while she was being treated in a hospital for a series of severe suicidal acts:

> I wind a thin wire around my limbs. Then I pull the wire tight till it slices through to the thigh bone. Then I lie on my back and bleed to death.

This dream occurred just after the return of her therapist from a vacation. Her associations included recalling that she used to help her father do electrical wiring around the house. She had struggled with her ambivalent feelings about extricating herself from the incestuous "tie" (another allusion to the wire), since she partly was horrified by what her father was doing and partly enjoyed the special bond of intimacy that the sexual behavior had fostered. In her view, the punishment for the taboo represented by the incest was death.

*   *   *

This dream was reported by a woman being treated on an inpatient unit. She had a mixed borderline and schizotypal personality disorder.

> I talk with someone from the hospital, but no one seems able to hear me, or at least they don't respond. The scene changes, and I am in a wintry setting. I fall in the snow and shout for help, but no one comes. I keep crying, "Help! Help!" but eventually I drown in the melted snow and die.

*   *   *

A young man with a mixed narcissistic and obsessional personality reported this dream. He functioned originally at the borderline level, though after some years of therapy he had progressed to a neurotic level. He had many first-degree relatives with various forms of manic-depressive illness.

> I play soccer with my brother. The players on the other side are mainly ruffians and "hoods." The hoods, after the game is over, kidnap my brother and then take me to an alley where President Ford is acting as a watchman or judge. As long as he is there, I feel safe, but when he turns his back for a moment, the hoods shoot me in the forehead, and I keel over dead. Later I wake up at home, with a hole in the back of my head and a piece of my head that's missing. There's blood all over me. I think I must be dying, and I call out to my parents. They don't hear me. I run to my girlfriend and tell her, "I'm dying!" Only she doesn't pay attention either.

This dream was apparently precipitated by a missed session necessitated by a change in schedule. The patient was also feeling nostalgic about a close friend, who happened to have the same name as his therapist. Inordinately attached to his mother, he used to talk with her for half an hour every night on the phone, even while he was in bed with his fiancée. This understandably infuriated his fiancée, who threatened to break off their relationship if he continued to engage in these protracted conversations in the middle of lovemaking. He feared alienating his mother if he cut short the conversations, and he feared losing his fiancée if he did not. Hence the fear, expressed in the dream, of losing both—a "fatal" consequence, given his dependency.

*   *   *

Patients with borderline structure are more liable than are normals and neurotics to have dreams of fragmentation, of being dead, of mutilation of their own body, and of naked aggression against the important persons in their life. These phenomena tend to be even more pronounced in psychotic patients, some of whom cannot even readily distinguish between the dream state and everyday reality.[2]

CONCLUSION

Dream analysis often provides better indications of the emotional factors at play with a borderline patient at any given moment than what the patient is aware of or is able to put into words. Paying attention to the dreams may help the therapist steer a more accurate course in deciding which dynamic is of paramount importance, and then in adhering to it, despite the diversionary tactics with which borderline patients so often baffle or confuse their therapists.

Therapists need to be aware, however, that borderline patients sometimes report dreams of seemingly endless length and infinite detail, consuming all but the last few minutes of the session with the reportage. Such patients are using their dreams primarily to conceal, not reveal, what is of importance in their lives at the time. By foreclosing any opportunity to work with the dream material, these patients are using the dream as a defense mechanism—specifically, as a peculiarity of communication (a pseudo-communication actually) that needs to be confronted and interpreted, much as one would with any other resistance.

---

[2]"Schizophrenics treat their dreams as though they were real experiences, and they confuse the content of their dreams with the products of their psychosis" (Erntz 1924, p. 292). Erntz adds that this is the case with only a portion of schizophrenic patients. His observations apply also to psychotic-level patients with delusional disorder. One such patient, whose delusional disorder took the form of erotomania, dreamed that the object of her love (a famous politician who had no acquaintance with her at all) was standing on a hill not far from her kitchen window, gazing fondly at her from a distance. To her this signified that he was really, albeit secretly, in love with her. This kind of distortion is not common with borderline patients, who are more apt to experience certain dreams as premonitory—foretelling with eerie accuracy what is about to happen.

The powerful transference emotions that characterize the therapeutic work with borderline patients are often particularly transparent in their dreams. The primitive nature of their dreams makes identification of the primary affects easier, even though the therapeutic work itself may be considerably stormier and more hazardous than is customarily the case with better integrated patients.

CHAPTER 12

Transference-Focused Psychotherapy Combined with Pharmacotherapy

With the success of pharmacologic agents in addressing specific symptoms in the Axis I disorders, investigators began empirical trials of these agents to treat similar symptoms in the personality disorder population. The conceptualization of borderline personality disorder first as a variant of schizophrenia and later as an affective disorder variant provided additional impetus for various medication trials. More recent evidence linking such borderline traits as impulsive aggression to serotonergic activity (Coccaro et al 1989), vulnerability to cognitive or perceptual distortion to dopaminergic activity, and affective instability to cholinergic or noradrenergic activity (Siever and Davis 1991) provided an additional theoretical rationale for pharmacotherapy in the treatment of personality disorders. Finally, patients with personality disorders may present with a concurrent Axis I disorder that responds to medication.

Although no single medication has emerged as the treatment of choice for borderline personality disorder, a number of agents have been shown to be effective for specific borderline symptoms. Medications also have important limitations and may complicate the treatment of borderline patients. Such central borderline features as the predominance of splitting, preoccupations with control of others and of being controlled, vulnerability to intense transference reactions, distortion of ordinary channels of communication to induce intense feelings in others, the potential for negative therapeutic reactions, and the induction of strong countertransferences make the use of medication in this population especially complicated. For these reasons, the decision to introduce medication must be carefully taken, and its use must be integrated with the overall treatment approach.

The psychodynamic psychotherapy of borderline patients may be terminated in its earliest phases, when borderline patients impulsively quit treatment in outbursts of anger. The emergence of affective storms during sessions may make it impossible for the patient to process the therapist's interventions and may make patient and therapist alike wary of evoking too much feeling in the hours. Vegetative depression may severely impair the patient's productivity in session, and psychotic regressions may threaten the ongoing treatment. To the extent that medications can address these intense symptoms, they may facilitate psychotherapy.

CURRENT EMPIRICAL FINDINGS

Although studies of the effectiveness of medication in the treatment of borderline personality disorder are complicated by a high placebo response, high dropout rates, and Axis I and II comorbidities, a number of findings have begun to emerge.

SELECTIVE SEROTONIN REUPTAKE INHIBITORS

Selective serotonin reuptake inhibitors (SSRIs) have been particularly attractive candidates for the treatment of borderline patients because of the association between decreased serotonergic activity and impulsive aggression and suicidal behavior; because these agents treat depression; and because they are relatively safe from the point of view of overdosage. Open-label trials of fluoxetine (Norden 1989) and sertraline (Kavoussi, Lin, and Cocarro 1994) have been promising but hard to interpret because of the high placebo responsiveness of borderline patients. Recently, Salzman and his colleagues (1995) conducted a twelve-week, randomized, placebo-controlled study of fluoxetine in twenty-seven relatively high-functioning, clinically diagnosed borderline patients recruited by newspaper advertisement. Patients received a mean dose of forty milligrams per day of active medication. There was a high improvement in the placebo group as well as in the drug group. However, fluoxetine was significantly superior to the placebo in reducing anger and depression. Five patients dropped out (19 percent). A note of caution in the use of SSRIs to treat borderline patients was raised by anecdotal reports of treatment-emergent violent suicidal ideation in depressed patients receiving fluoxetine. A subsequent study by Mann and Kapur (1991) suggests that this response is infrequent, affecting fewer than 5 percent of patients, and is unlikely to be specific to the SSRIs as opposed to other antidepressants.

MONOAMINE OXIDASE INHIBITORS

Liebowitz and Klein (1981) proposed using the monoamine oxidase inhibitor (MOAI) phenelzine to treat a group of rejection-sensitive patients he called "hysteroid dysphorics." In a drug discontinuation design, they treated sixteen hysteroid dysphorics, twelve of whom met *DSM-III* criteria for BPD, with fifteen to seventy-five milligrams per day of phenelzine for three months, and then blindly switched six of the remaining patients to a placebo for the next three months. All patients received twice-weekly psychodynamic psychotherapy. During the initial three-month open-label phase, there was significant improvement in depression, anxiety, affective lability, and specific features related to rejection sensitivity. Among the six switched to a placebo, four worsened when they were off the active medication. Thirty-one percent of the patients dropped out within the first four months.

In an elegant placebo-controlled crossover design, Cowdry and Gardner (1988) studied six-week trials of four medications in treating *DSM-III* BPD patients who had serious behavioral dyscontrol and met Klein's criteria for hysteroid dysphoria. Subjects agreed to remain in psychotherapy for the duration of the drug study. Cowdry and Gardner found that tranylcypromine (at a mean dose of forty milligrams per day) was superior to the placebo in decreasing impulsivity, anger, suicidality, rejection sensitivity, and depression. Although the overall effect of tranylcypromine was positive and it was highly rated by patients, some caution may be warranted: a subgroup of three of the twelve patients receiving the drug demonstrated severe behavioral dyscontrol. One-quarter of the patients in the tranylcypromine group dropped out of treatment. Soloff and his colleagues (1993) conducted a placebo-controlled, randomized trial of phenelzine (with an average dose of sixty milligrams per day) and low-dose haloperidol (average dose of four milligrams per day) over a five-week period in an initially hospitalized group of borderline patients. They reported that phenelzine was superior to the placebo in reducing depression, anger, hostility, anxiety, and the overall number of borderline symptoms. The attrition rate in the phenelzine group was 24 percent. They report that time and milieu treatment was also effective in reducing symptoms, particularly depressive symptoms. Addressing the lack of information about the effects of medication in borderline patients beyond the five- to twelve-week trials in most studies, Soloff's group (Cornelius et al. 1993) followed this same cohort of patients for an additional sixteen weeks. They found that over this longer time period phenelzine demonstrated only modest efficacy in treating depression and irritability.

Mood Stabilizers / Anticonvulsants

In their six-week crossover study, Cowdry and Gardner (1988) found the anticonvulsant and mood stabilizer carbamezepine (at a mean daily dose of 820 milligrams) to be superior to the placebo in physician-rated improvement in impulsivity, suicidality, anger, anxiety, euphoria, and overall symptomatology. The dropout rate was 33 percent. Sodium valproate, another anticonvulsant and mood stabilizer, showed promise in a small open-label study (Stein et al. 1995). Three of eleven patients could not complete the eight-week trial. Among the completers, four showed improvement in overall pathology and mood, and three improved in the areas of impulsivity, subjective irritability, anger, anxiety, and rejection sensitivity. Links and his colleagues (1990) compared lithium (at a mean dose of 986 milligrams per day) and desipramine (mean dose of 168 milligrams per day) in a six-week, double-blind, placebo-controlled, random-order, crossover design in the treatment of nineteen borderline patients. They found a trend for lithium to be superior to desipramine and the placebo in the reduction of anger and suicidality. Therapists rated lithium as significantly superior to the placebo, but patients did not. In an open-label trial of the anticonvulsant lamotrigine, Pinto and Akiskal (1998) reported a dramatic response in three of eight BPD patients at doses of 75 to 300 milligrams per day, with a mean improvement in a global assessment of functioning (GAF) score from the 40s to the 80s over a three- to four-month period. One patient was discontinued because of a rash, one dropped out, and the remaining three failed on lamotrigine but responded to sertraline, valproate, and lithium-thioridizine combination, respectively.

LOW-DOSE NEUROLEPTICS

A number of studies have shown that low doses of neuroleptics (for example, four to eight milligrams of haloperidol, eight milligrams of trifluoperazine, or nine milligrams of thiothixene) are superior to a placebo in reducing anxiety and such quasi-psychotic symptoms in borderline patients as ideas of reference, illusions, and cognitive disturbances (Goldberg et al. 1986; Soloff et al. 1989; Cowdry and Gardner 1988). Montgomery (1987), Cowdry and Gardner (1988), and Soloff and his colleagues (1989) also reported that low doses of neuroleptics reduced suicidality and impulsivity in borderline patients. Two studies (Cowdry and Gardener 1988; Soloff et al. 1989) report that low-dose neuroleptics reduce interpersonal sensitivity and depression. Two other studies (Goldberg et al. 1986; Soloff et al. 1993) do not find a significant effect on depression. Soloff's group, which had initially reported that a broad spectrum of borderline symptoms responded to haloperidol in a five-week trial, was not able to replicate this response in a second sample of borderline inpatients, perhaps because the second sample had fewer quasi-psychotic symptoms at baseline (Soloff 1994). In their sixteen-week continuation trial, Soloff and his colleagues (Cornelius et al. 1993) found that haloperidol remained effective over this period only in reducing irritability.

TRICYCLIC ANTIDEPRESSANTS AND ANXIOLYTICS

Borderline patients are often prescribed tricyclic antidepressants to address persistent depressive symptoms, but the work of Soloff's group (Soloff et al. 1989) brings this practice into question. They found that 58 percent of the borderline inpatients in the sample showed a worsening in hostile depression, and 64 percent a worsening in schizotypal symptoms, on a five-week trial of amitriptlyene. Because of their disinhibitory effect and addictive potential, benzodiazepines should be used with great caution in borderline patients. Cowdry and Gardner (1988) reported significantly higher suicidality among patients treated with alprazolam than among those receiving a placebo.

OVERVIEW OF PSYCHOPHARMACOLOGIC FINDINGS

The drug studies have shown that borderline patients respond to a variety of psychiatric medications, with different constellations of symptoms preferentially responding to different medications, although there is some overlap. No single medication appears to be the drug of choice for BPD (Soloff 1994). The results of efforts to use differential response to various medications as a means of dissecting BPD into subsyndromes have thus far not lived up to expectations (Soloff et al. 1993). The state of the art in medicating borderline patients is to select a medication on the basis of the most prominent symptoms:

- Tranylcypromine, carbamazepine, low-dose neuroleptics, or possibly SSRIs for impulsivity, suicidality, and self-directed aggression
- SSRIs, MAOIs, low-dose neuroleptics, carbamazepine, and possibly valproate for excessive anger
- MAOIs and SSRIs for depression
- Lithium for mood swings
- MAOIs for rejection sensitivity
- Low-dose neuroleptics for referential thinking, paranoid ideation, derealization, and perceptual distortions

Table 12.1 summarizes the medications that can be expected to treat acutely each borderline symptom complex, based on the findings of placebo-controlled studies or, where no controlled studies are available, open-label studies that are consistent with a theoretical model. Because of the potential for dangerous tyramine reactions to MAOIs, caution should be taken in prescribing them to unreliable patients. Since it is difficult to predict in advance which patient will respond to which medication, a sequential trial of two or three medications may be necessary to obtain an optimal result (Stein 1992).

Although pharmacologic studies have demonstrated effects that are statistically significant, the magnitude of improvement is generally modest—symptoms typically improve from "severe" to "moderate" on rating scales. In addition, the duration of medication effect is uncertain: most studies have lasted only five to twelve weeks, and one longer continuation study suggested a diminution in effectiveness of both haloperidol and phenelzine by

TABLE 12-1   Medications for Symptom Complexes in Borderline Patients

Symptom Pattern	SSRIs	Carbamazepine	Valproate	Lithium	Low-Dose Neuroleptic	MAO Inhibitor
Impulsivity, suicidality	X	X			X	X
Excessive anger	X	X	X		X	X
Depression	X					X
Rejection sensitivity						X
Mood swings				X		
Cognitive-perceptual					X	

the twenty-first week (Cornelius et al. 1993). The medication studies have also confirmed that many borderline patients show significant improvement from the impact of a therapeutic milieu or simply the placebo effect. An additional limitation to the effectiveness of pharmacotherapy is the high medication discontinuation rate.

COMBINED TREATMENT

THEORETICAL RATIONALE

Since psychotherapy and pharmacotherapy have specific areas of strength and weakness in treating borderline patients, it is reasonable to consider combining them, particularly for patients who have not responded to one modality alone. Medication appears to have its maximal effectiveness early, while psychotherapy may take longer to produce change. Psychotherapy and medication both reduce self-destructive behavior, but depressive moods may not be alleviated during the early phase of psychotherapy and may respond to medication sooner, especially vegetative depressions. Cognitive distortions, which can impede psychotherapy, may be reduced by low-dose neuroleptics. Finally, although both psychotherapy and pharmacotherapy have high dropout rates, together they may work synergistically to reduce premature terminations. Borderline patients typically discontinue treatment in the first few months because of their anger and impulsivity (Smith et al. 1995). SSRIs, MAOIs, carbamezepine, and low-dose neuroleptics have been shown to reduce these symptoms. On the other hand, borderline patients may also discontinue medication because of an overreaction to side effects, unaddressed transference reactions to the pharmacologist, and distorted meanings attributed to the medication or to the experience of "being medicated." Concurrent psychotherapy provides an opportunity to defuse these issues.

Although combined treatment is very promising across a wide range of clinical conditions, there are many potential complications. The use of combined treatment with borderline patients is especially complicated by the effects of splitting, omnipotent control, intense transference reactions, rejection sensitivity, affective instability, and impulsivity. When the therapist makes a recommendation to add medication or psychotherapy, specific reactions of the borderline patient to the recommended modality will influence the treatment process and the processes special to these patients will be activated.

SOME CONSEQUENCES OF INTRODUCING MEDICATION

When medication is brought to the psychotherapeutic setting, meanings that the patient associates with the medication will color the psychotherapeutic process and affect medication compliance. Because of the preponderance of defenses like omnipotent control and projective identification, the borderline patient is often preoccupied with fears of being controlled and with efforts to be in control. Medication may be seen in this context as a means by which the therapist is attempting to gain control over the patient's mind. This may lead to power struggles around medication—medication refusals, control of dosing, demands for more medication. Medication may be experienced as an extension of the physician who prescribes it. When the therapist is seen as a bad object, his prescription is likely to be perceived as toxic. On the other hand, patients may ingest medication to incorporate a "good" therapist. Medication may serve as a transitional object when confronting separations from the therapist.

Patients may consider medication as drugs with abuse potential and become concerned that they will become addicted. Patients who have strong dependent traits in particular may experience a therapist's prescription of medication as an effort to "hook" them on a drug and thus make them dependent on the therapist. Such patients often ask the therapist whether they will ever be able to stop the medication or whether it is addicting.

The therapist's act of prescribing medication in the context of a psychotherapeutic relationship may also have special meaning to the patient. It may be experienced as an act of desperation by the therapist: convinced that psychotherapy is failing, the therapist is resorting to medication in a last-ditch effort. The introduction of medication may also be seen as an effort by the therapist to distance himself from the patient.

SOME CONSEQUENCES OF INTRODUCING PSYCHOTHERAPY

Just as medication and its prescription may have individualized meanings to the patient, so too does the recommendation of psychotherapy. For patients in whom dependency conflicts prevail, the suggestion that they come one or more times a week may be seen itself as an effort to make them dependent on the therapist. In patients with strong narcissistic pathology or antisocial features, the recommendation of frequent sessions may be seen as an exploitation, a way to make money at the patient's expense. Patients may also see the recommendation of psychotherapy as a seduction. With Freud linked in the popular culture to the notion of sexuality, patients fearing a seduction sometimes express this by asking the therapist simply, "Are you a Freudian?" To some, the need for psychotherapy signals that, rather than suffering from an acceptable illness, they have a weakness in character. If they were strong enough, they would not need a psychotherapist. Finally, the introduction of regular psychotherapy into a primarily psychopharmacologic treatment can be expected to intensify the transference.

SPECIAL COMPLICATIONS ARISING OUT OF BORDERLINE PATHOLOGY

The defense of splitting, in which borderline patients maintain starkly opposite representations of themselves and others, leads to special complications when medication is combined with psychotherapy. The use of medication implies a conceptualization of the patient's illness as biologically mediated, while a psychotherapeutic approach implies that psychological processes underlie the illness. Although the therapist may appreciate that personality symptoms sometimes respond to both talking and biological treatments, borderline patients view the treatment in an either-or manner. When medication and psychotherapy are used together, the patient may alternate between a biological and psychological sense of self. One representation may be used to defend against the other when anxiety threatens.

For example, Miss B., a woman with BPD, was being treated with an MAOI for a comorbid atypical depression. She would defend against invitations to examine her emotional reactions to events in her life to better understand her mood shifts by attributing them solely to her menstrual cycle. When the therapist confronted her avoidance, she responded that it was clear that her moods could be understood on a biochemical basis without recourse to understanding her psychological reactions because she had been helped by an antidepressant.

Borderline patients are especially prone to act, rather than feel conflict or anxiety. They act to influence the feelings and behavior of others as they employ such defenses as omnipotent control and projective identification. Medication is often a convenient vehicle for the borderline patient's acting out. Patients may seek to induce anxiety in the therapist by stockpiling medications, taking dangerous risks in regulating the dose themselves, combining medications with alcohol, violating an MAOI diet, or using medication in a suicide gesture or attempt. When prescribed medication becomes a preferred method for suicide attempts and the patient cannot be trusted to contract for safety, the use of medication may be contraindicated.

Psychotherapeutic work with borderline patients typically entails strong countertransference feelings, often induced in the therapist by the patient's use of projective identification. Like the patients themselves, the therapists of borderline patients can be induced to enact unconscious feelings. The opportunity for the therapist to act in regulating medication may become an avenue for countertransference enactments. Maltsberger and Buie (1974) have described the phenomenon of hate in the countertransference toward suicidal patients. The prescription of tricyclic antidepressants to a borderline patient reporting suicidal depression could represent an unconscious collusion: it would place into the hands of an acutely suicidal individual a potentially lethal agent that takes weeks to have any antidepressant effect.

The negative therapeutic reaction is another complicating factor in the combined treatment of borderline patients. Freud described this reaction as a paradoxical worsening of the patient following good therapeutic work. He suggested that it arose from unconscious guilt. With borderline patients, a negative therapeutic reaction may develop from intense envy of the therapist's capacity to help: the patient obtains gratification from defeating the therapist. Borderline patients may also show negative therapeutic reactions because they can relate to the therapist only by fusing their affection with their sadism. We have discussed in chapters 5 and 9 that such negative therapeutic reactions are often seen in patients who fall on the narcissistic-antisocial spectrum and in patients who suffered early sexual abuse. In the psychopharmacologic sphere, negative therapeutic reaction may take the form of the patient discontinuing medication at the first sign that it is helping.

ASSESSING THE NEED
FOR COMBINED TREATMENT

The combination of medication and psychotherapy may be extremely valuable for some borderline patients, but many patients with this diagnosis are best treated with psychotherapy alone, and others with pharmacotherapy alone. Psychotherapy is usually an important element in the treatment of borderline patients because it fosters the examination of the interpersonal relationships and self representations that are the source of much of their distress. In some cases, however, psychotherapy is contraindicated (Frances and Clarkin 1981). Although negative therapeutic reactions can usually be surmounted by confronting them and interpreting their origins and functions, this is not always the case. For some borderline patients, as treatment progresses, negative therapeutic reactions lead to increasingly dangerous symptoms. For these patients, no treatment is the treatment of choice, unless an acute, life-saving intervention is called for. Chronically dependent patients for whom the pleasures of being in psychotherapy take precedence over recovery, because of the gratifications of ongoing contact with a therapist, may also benefit from a period without psychotherapy. If the indications for pharmacotherapy are present, these patients may be candidates for a solely pharmacologic treatment with infrequent and brief meetings. For most borderline patients, however, the question is whether pharmacotherapy should be added to psychotherapy.

In making this assessment, the therapist first considers whether there is a comorbid condition known to respond to medication. Thus, in the presence of major depression, bipolar disorder, obsessive-compulsive disorder, or adult attention deficit disorder, pharmacotherapy would be instituted to treat the Axis I condition. Medical disorders that might produce psychiatric symptoms, such as seizure disorders and endocrinopathies, should be considered and treated medically as appropriate. In addressing such borderline symptoms as impulsivity, suicidality, anger, psychoticism, affective instability, rejection sensitivity, and depression, medications are most helpful in the more severely symptomatic patients. As in all pharmacologic assessments, the history of response to prior medication trials may be a useful guide. Inquiry into the patient's experience of side effects with medications is valuable not only for the selection of medication but also as an indicator of potential compliance difficulties. Medication may be contraindicated if there is a history of severe acting out with medications, such as the stockpiling of medications for suicide attempts or the use of medication to derail the treatment by exclusively focusing on somatic issues. When the initial evaluation is conducted by a psychiatrist, the pharmacotherapeutic evaluation is carried out at the same time. If the evaluator is a nonphysician, he or she refers the patient for a psychopharmacologic consultation.

ONE THERAPIST OR TWO?

Is combined treatment of the borderline patient best carried out by a single psychiatrist, or by a psychotherapist and a psychopharmacologist working together? Each model has its advantages and drawbacks. An important advantage of the single-therapist model is that it minimizes the countertherapeutic effects of splitting. As mentioned earlier, the introduction of medication creates a cleavage line for splits between biological and psychological self representations. When the treatment is divided between therapists who signify each side of the split, it is more difficult to address this defense. The presence of two therapists also provides opportunities for the patient to play out internal contradictions by inducing actual conflict between the therapists (by means of projective identification or omnipotent control). Such externalized conflicts can be quite destructive to treatment. Finally, the dual-therapist model introduces the complications of divided lines of authority and responsibility.

A single-therapist model avoids these complexities but raises its own complications. Pharmacological treatment and psychotherapy have different role requirements for the therapist. The pharmacotherapist is generally quite directive, inquiring about changes in target symptoms, asking about specific side effects, directing dosage changes, ordering blood tests, and performing parts of a physical examination. The psychotherapist, on the other hand, particularly in exploratory psychotherapy, observes as the patient sets the agenda for the session, refrains from interrupting the flow, minimizes instructions to the patient, and avoids physically examining the patient. Nevertheless, it is possible for a single psychiatrist to conduct a combined treatment if the treatment is structured to contain both modalities. Thus, a specific time is reserved for medication issues—for example, the first fifteen minutes of the first session of the week. Symptom changes and side effects are elicited, and prescriptions are written. When medication issues expand beyond this frame or invade other portions of the treatment, the therapist is alerted to consider whether they reflect defensive, transference, or countertransference processes. Of course, important drug reactions may arise at any time, and the therapist must address them as needed.

When a psychopharmacologist and psychotherapist collaborate under the dual-therapist model, they must specify in advance who will take responsibility for the decision to hospitalize and who will be called for crises. The model works best when the therapists are familiar with each other's work, share a common conceptual frame of reference, and communicate regularly about the patient. Regularly scheduled discussions are preferable to as-needed conferences because they enhance the collaborative relationship, keep the treatment coordinated, and, most important, allow incipient splits in the treatment to be identified at the earliest opportunity.

Case Examples of Combined Treatment

The following cases illustrate more fully how psychodynamically motivated themes interact with practical pharmacologic issues in combined treatment. Illustrations are drawn from both single-therapist and dual-therapist models.

Using the Single-Therapist Model in the Psychotherapeutic Process to Address Medication Noncompliance.   Miss A., who was receiving twice-weekly psychodynamic psychotherapy and concurrent antidepressant medication, began her forty-fourth session by announcing a unilateral decision to discontinue the medication and not to complete a research questionnaire required as a precondition for her treatment.

The discussion of these refusals elicited Miss A.'s feelings about the therapist. She saw him as cruelly controlling and as having threatened to end the treatment unless she complied with the research requirements. She felt compelled either to submit to the therapist or to be deprived of something essential. She went on to express a fantasy about the medication: she believed the medication controlled her by "subduing" a part of her.

Thus, Miss A. experienced herself in the transference as a powerless victim in relation to a therapist who sought to control her to further his own interests at her expense. Recalling that she had expressed rather different feelings about him during a recent session, the therapist confronted Miss A. by juxtaposing these two contradictory transference configurations: "In some ways it sounds as if my taking a stance in this issue has confirmed for you a perception that in fact I shouldn't be trusted with your welfare and that I don't have your interests at heart." Miss A. agreed, and the therapist continued: she believed, he said, that he "would actually do something harmful to you just to benefit someone else. . . . That's very different, though, from the ideas you've expressed today, and recently you've said, in fact, [that] you feel I'm trustworthy and ethical. This idea is just the opposite, that in fact I'm really not." Miss A. acknowledged having both views of the therapist. As the session ended, the therapist wondered about the contradiction and asked Miss A. whether she were curious about it too.

When Miss A. arrived at the next session, she announced that she had resumed the medication. She reported that she had realized that the therapist might have had her best interests in mind after all and that she did not need to struggle with him so much for control.

This example illustrates a way to address medication noncompliance through direct work with the transference. A confrontation helped the patient become temporarily better integrated and undercut an acting-out that involved medication noncompliance.

The Dual-Therapist Model: Collaboration Between Therapists and Transference to the Pharmacotherapist.   Ms. C., a fifty-two-year-old professor of English, was referred for a medication consultation by a clinical psychologist colleague. Ms. C. had presented with the complaint that suicide had begun to make logical sense to her; she wanted to see whether therapy could shed some light on this conviction before she took action. If she did take action, it would be either by shooting herself with an antique pistol she owned or by taking an overdose. Ms. C. had been undergoing treatment for a chronic medical condition and had recently been told of a new complication.

In a telephone conversation, arranged before the psychiatrist's first meeting with Ms. C., the psychotherapist described her as quite intelligent, with a wry and biting wit; she was a patient whose charm, altruism, and self-deprecatory humor made her quite likable, in spite of her tendency toward bitterness and her strong narcissistic features. She reported a repetitive theme in her important relationships: being taken by surprise by sudden betrayals and abandonments by others. The consultation was sought to determine whether an antidepressant was indicated for the depression. The psychologist began once-a-week sessions with Ms. C.

The psychopharmacologist saw Ms. C. for a consultation and obtained a full psychiatric and medical history. He diagnosed a major depression and a borderline personality organization with a narcissistic personality. He felt that Ms. C. was not acutely suicidal, but because of the severity of the depressive symptoms, he prescribed an SSRI during the first visit. He telephoned the referring psychologist to inform him that he had started medication, to share impressions, and to review the risk of suicide. Both therapists shared a similar view of the patient. The psychotherapist would continue to see Ms. C. weekly in psychodynamic psychotherapy, and the psychiatrist would see her weekly at first, to initiate the antidepressant treatment, and then with decreasing frequency.

At Ms. C.'s second visit to the pharmacotherapist one week later, there was little change. On the third visit, three weeks after beginning the medication, she reported an improvement in the depression, decreased anhedonia, improved sleep, and less worry about suicide. She also reported a "free-floating" anger that began on the afternoon of the visit to the pharmacotherapist. When the pharmacologist wondered whether this was related to her feelings about the visit, Ms. C. said that she doubted it. She reported that she felt positive about her work with the psychotherapist and was continuing to see him weekly. He said they were beginning to look at her dreams.

At the next visit, one month later, Ms. C. reported that the depressive symptoms continued to improve, but she spoke of anxiety about an upcoming medical procedure. In the last moments of the session, she asked for a benzodiazepine for sleep. Because there was no time to examine the request in that session and to identify possible psychological factors in the insomnia, the pharmacotherapist suggested that Ms. C. discuss this problem with her psychotherapist and call for another appointment if she continued to feel the need for sleep medication; otherwise, they would meet in two months. This illustrates one approach to the end-of-session request. Borderline patients often "act in" by raising an important issue in the final moments of a session when there is no time for exploration. In regular psychotherapy, such issues can usually be referred to the next session, and their emergence at the very last minute can also be examined. This is not possible with infrequent pharmacotherapy meetings, so the pharmacologist directs further examination of the psychological aspects of the request to the psychotherapy and offers an earlier appointment if separate medication issues remain.

Ms. C. did not request an extra pharmacotherapy session but returned for the scheduled appointment two months later. She asked whether the SSRI could be wearing off: She was beginning to feel more depressed. She mentioned, in passing, that her therapist was on vacation and that she was feeling stress about her own upcoming vacation. The pharmacotherapist suggested that these factors might be contributing to the depression and suggested watchful waiting rather than an increase in medication. When reminded of her request for a benzodiazepine in the last session, Ms. C. reported that she had used it in the past for sleep and also to treat public speaking anxiety. Her next association was to the "writer's block" that she was discussing with her psychotherapist.

Ms. C. continued in her regular psychotherapy but canceled her next pharmacotherapy session and rescheduled it so that she was next seen four months after her last appointment. At that session, she reported that her mood continued to be good, she was able to enjoy herself, and sleep and appetite were good. She reported that she had been dreaming a good deal. She spoke of a dream in which a cab driver was about to take her along a dangerous route through a park at night, but she insisted on getting out of the cab at a public square where a large monument stood. She felt this dream symbolized her recognition that she had renounced suicide as an option. She said her therapist had interpreted it as a dream about the therapy. She then related a dream in which she was delayed on an important mission by the need to see a particular novelist. When the pharmacotherapist asked whether Ms. C. was aware that this author's original family name was the same as that of the pharmacotherapist, Ms. C. said that she was, and then went on to speak of her resentment about having to see a pharmacotherapist and a psychotherapist. Here the pharmacotherapist intervened with the dream material because it appeared to reflect a transference to him, and the cancellation of the previous session had already raised in her mind the possibility that a negative transference might be threatening the continuation of the dual treatment. Ms. C.'s response confirmed this hypothesis and permitted the negative feelings to be discussed openly. No further exploration of the sources of this resentment was attempted. Ms. C.'s depressive symptoms remained in good control, and she continued her regular psychotherapy and kept her bimonthly pharmacotherapy appointments.

Fifteen months after the beginning of treatment, the psychotherapist telephoned the pharmacotherapist to tell him that Ms. C. had decided to interrupt psychotherapy for financial reasons that the therapist felt were realistic. He asked whether the pharmacotherapist were willing to continue seeing Ms. C. for pharmacotherapy alone. Both therapists felt this was appropriate. In the next pharmacotherapy session, Ms. C. discussed her decision to interrupt the psychotherapy and asked to continue the pharmacotherapy.

This development raises an issue that not uncommonly arises in dual treatment—the decision to stop one part of the treatment. The initial contract for a dual treatment should make it clear that the pharmacotherapy is available only as part of a combined treatment. This reduces the likelihood that the patient will enact a split in which one therapist is seen as all good and retained, and the other as all bad and rejected. Of course, there are times when continuing one limb of the treatment is appropriate. The wish to terminate one portion of the treatment should be carefully explored by both therapists, and they should decide together on an appropriate recommendation to make to the patient. Ms. C.'s psychotherapist felt that the realistic factors made the psychotherapy interruption appropriate, but it is also possible that the issue related to seeing two doctors that emerged when the dream was examined had not been adequately explored and contributed to the interruption.

This case, presented from the point of view of the pharmacotherapist, illustrates a low-intensity collaboration in the treatment of a high-functioning borderline patient. During the treatment, each therapist consistently conveyed support for the importance of the other modality by expressing interest in the patient's work with the other therapist. Transference phenomena surfaced in the pharmacotherapeutic sessions as well as in the exploratory sessions and were explored by the pharmacotherapist to a limited extent—that is, only when they appeared to signal a possible strain in their alliance.

*   *   *

A combined psychotherapeutic-psychopharmacologic approach can enhance the treatment of some borderline patients with comorbid Axis I conditions or of those with significant levels of impulsivity, anger, self-directed aggression, or perceptual-cognitive symptoms. It requires careful attention to the psychological meanings of the treatment components, the complications introduced by the primitive defenses, the coordination of the therapist and pharmacotherapist roles, and the emerging transference and countertransference themes.

CHAPTER 13

Transference-Focused Psychotherapy in Sequence with Other Modalities

It is characteristic of patients with borderline personality disorder to have a succession of different kinds of treatment over the course of their lifetime, often beginning in childhood or adolescence, when problems begin to surface for many of them. Family and friends, unable to tolerate or understand their unhappiness and kaleidoscopic behavior, become puzzled, disappointed, and enraged by the inconsistency between the intelligence of some of these children, on the one hand, and their unreasonableness and emotionality, on the other, or between their apparently fortunate circumstances and the extremes of their unhappiness.

THE LIFE TRAJECTORY OF MULTIPLE COURSES OF TREATMENT IN BPD

The history of adult patients diagnosed as borderline therefore not uncommonly includes a period of psychotherapy or psychoanalysis in childhood or adolescence. Skillful treatment may serve to help the patient through a critical period while some concomitant developmental increase in ego strength enables the negotiation of subsequent challenges—until the challenges of young adulthood overtax the patient's emotional resources.

CASE EXAMPLES

Two patients, one a nine-year-old boy analyzed during a four-year period of hospitalization, the other a thirteen-year-old girl analyzed for two years as an outpatient, presented with borderline personality organization and behavioral symptoms whose severity exceeded the parents' capacity to manage them. Both showed behavioral improvement over the course of treatment. When seen several years after termination, when both were in their early twenties, the original borderline personality structure was found to have been succeeded by the consolidation of a narcissistic personality that clearly would compromise the patients' interpersonal and vocational progress. Neither patient, however, saw a need for treatment at that point.

As young adults, borderline patients typically respond to the normal developmental challenge of finding partners and establishing careers with a new awareness that they lack a sense of self, a growing sense of failure, and feelings of despair. At this point, they may embark on self-destructive behavior in the attempt to manage the profound anxiety associated with the feelings of emptiness that bespeak their identity diffusion. They are often referred for hospitalization in the wake of threats or attempts of suicide. In the past, such hospitalizations were often lengthy; today the typical pattern is one of frequent, brief hospitalizations, with attempts at pharmacological management of symptoms. The histories of older patients often include accounts of protracted periods in hospitals, with variable outcomes. A study of such cases (Stone 1990) suggests that hospitalizations tended to have a favorable effect on the subsequent course of illness.

Patients whose symptomatology includes self-mutilating or addictive behavior, minor criminality, or chronic interpersonal or vocational failures tend to find their way to outpatient treatments of various kinds, usually beginning with attempts at supportive psychotherapy that may go on for many years. Extended periods of supportive psychotherapy may reflect an ongoing helpful alliance; in some cases, unfortunately, such therapy reflects the development of hostile dependency or of an exploitive relationship that recapitulates abuse the patient experienced in early life.

Ms. L. harbored an enduring sense of being entitled to reclaim a childhood that had been spoiled by her "parentification" by severely compromised parents. As a young adult, she impoverished her parents through endless expensive treatments, including hospitalizations precipitated by suicide attempts. Supportive psychotherapy ended after many years when the therapist became exhausted by her threats, demands, and lack of progress.

This case illustrates the typical sequence of a trial of supportive psychotherapy or psychoanalysis to which the patient responds either with no change or with escalating self-destructive behaviors, culminating in a succession of hospitalizations and a therapist who has reached the limit of willingness to continue the attempt at treatment. At this point, the patient may be referred for evaluation as to the suitability of TFP as the next level of intervention.

Another common sequence, typical of the many patients who were abused and neglected in childhood, is one in which the illness goes unrecognized or is ignored until a suicide attempt precipitates hospitalization; the patient's subsequent failure to respond to ordinary hospital and outpatient treatment leads to consideration of TFP. In a third sequence, a patient is seen as a candidate for psychoanalysis but experiences severe exacerbation of symptoms in analytic treatment. The analyst introduces supportive elements into the treatment, but the deterioration cannot be stemmed; the patient is hospitalized and eventually referred for TFP. Or the analyst may restructure the treatment as TFP and so establish a workable relationship.

The suffering of these patients, combined with their readiness to experience treatment as futile, harmful, disappointing, or excessively demanding, often leads to many fits and starts, changes of therapists, and attempts at various forms of both conventional and alternative forms of therapy. It is thus against a background of many treatment failures that borderline patients tend to be referred for transference-focused psychotherapy. It is the rare case when the initial consultant sees TFP as the first and definitive approach to treatment of a borderline patient, as TFP remains a relatively new and controversial modality and trained practitioners are in short supply. Furthermore, TFP requires an unusually explicit and serious commitment on the part of the prospective patient. For these and various other reasons having to do with theoretical, ideological, and attitudinal leanings on the part of patients and clinicians, transference-focused psychotherapy is often seen as a treatment of last resort.

PREPARATORY TREATMENTS TO TFP

Even when TFP is clearly indicated, patients vary in their readiness to undertake it; some require a period of preparatory treatment in order to maximize the likelihood of benefiting from TFP. Preparatory treatments include hospitalization, medication, a course of cognitive-behavioral, group, and/or family therapy, vocational counseling or job training, and treatment of severe eating disorders or substance abuse. Some of these interventions may have to be continued as adjuncts to TFP until the latter is well established.

PSYCHOANALYSIS SUBSEQUENT TO TFP

TFP has a clear goal and an identifiable end point. It is specifically designed to bring about an integration of the part-objects that populate the patient's inner world and of the incompatible, unconscious object relations that account for the identity diffusion and behavioral fragmentation from which these patients suffer. The subsiding of flagrantly destructive and self-destructive behavior seen relatively early in the course of successful TFP does not signify such integration but rather a combination of dependence on the therapist and the therapy, fantasies of being rejected for "breaches" of the treatment contract, a developing interest in the interaction with the therapist, and growing recognition of the aggressive intent of the pathological behaviors and of the seriousness of the illness. As interpretive work goes on in the context of decreasing destructive behavior outside the therapy and increasing awareness of feelings of hatred, fear, and envy within the therapy, self and object representations begin to be integrated. Such integration is manifest in patients' occasional explicit statements such as, "I'm beginning to have a conscience," or, "I can see now the effect my illness has had on the people who love me." It is manifest as well when patients begin to be able to work or study consistently, to maintain relationships, to feel genuinely responsible for the ongoing course of their lives, and to experience genuine and appropriate guilt, gratitude, and mourning. At this stage, the original fragmentation of the inner world of the patient can be said to have been replaced by a consistent ego ideal and an organized ego, into which identifications with the therapist and other valued objects of desire and aggressive strivings have been absorbed. When the mosaic of conflicting, unconscious object relations has been replaced by an intrapsychic structure of an integrated ego and superego, and when the pattern of defenses has changed from reliance on splitting and its associated defensive operations to one organized around repression, TFP has fulfilled its mandate. At this point, either termination or referral for psychoanalysis is indicated.

A case example illustrates one aspect of integration: the stepwise process of moving from internalizing a part-object to identification with the self-reflective function of the therapist. A ten-year-old boy, after a year of treatment, reported that when his mind was awhirl he could calm himself by shouting inwardly, "I'm in therapy!", thus reminding himself of the existence of the therapist as a lifeline, however tenuous. Later he said that when he felt upset he would talk to himself "just like a therapist," suggesting idealization and imitation as an early stage of internalization. Still later he built a model bridge and said it was a bridge between himself and the therapist—"a bridge over troubled waters" that acknowledged the value of the therapeutic relationship. Finally, at age thirteen, he said, "When I'm upset I meditate, and usually I can figure things out for myself without having to talk with you about it." Identification with the interpretive function seemed to have been achieved.

When reliance on splitting and projection has given way to the flexible use of defensive operations, and when reduction of hatred and envy has permitted helpful identifications to be formed, the patient is capable of intensifying the therapy without pathological regression or overinvolvement in the treatment to the neglect of other important aspects of life. If there is evidence at this juncture of intrapsychic conflict that interferes with the realization of the patient's potential for creativity and happiness, psychoanalysis may be the appropriate next phase of treatment.

POST-TERMINATION "BOOSTER" SESSIONS

It is desirable to terminate TFP when the integrative work has been accomplished. Usually by this time patients are well advised to focus on their work and their interpersonal relationships as part of what has been an ongoing process of loosening their dependence on the therapist. Identification with the interpretive and affect-regulating functions of the therapist may be sufficiently solid to sustain the patient in ordinary daily functioning, but the occasional meeting of patient and therapist to consider a life crisis, to reflect on an important pending decision, or to deal with grief or disappointment may serve to shore up the crucial identification with the ego functions of the therapist or to validate and strengthen the gains the patient has made. Such sessions will be of a primarily interpretive or primarily supportive nature, as indicated.

IDENTIFYING PATIENTS WHO NEED PREPARATORY TREATMENT

The initial assessment process is crucial in determining whether TFP is indicated for a particular patient and, if not, whether some other form of treatment might be helpful. Some patients who have failed to respond to various other forms of treatment clearly need and could benefit from transference-focused psychotherapy. That is, they have the requisite intelligence, they have actual or potential social supports, and they fulfill the criteria for the diagnosis of borderline personality organization. But among such candidates for TFP are some whose failure to respond to other modalities is attributable to an antisocial character structure that will prove immune to any psychotherapeutic intervention. Preparatory treatment is futile in such cases. Others show a combination of symptoms and character structure that makes fruitful participation in TFP highly unlikely unless preceded by or combined with other modalities. Typical of the latter problems are cases of addiction or, broadly speaking, an entire spectrum of "cravings." Other patients who may require treatment in another modality as preparation for TFP include those whose high anxiety, combined with impoverished coping skills and an unsupportive or toxic social setting, renders them unable and unwilling to tolerate the treatment framework in which TFP is carried out. The interval of two to five days between the twice-weekly sessions and the avoidance of such supportive measures as between-session telephone calls or participation in the patient's daily life decisions can tax the resources of such patients beyond their limit, necessitating a course of supportive or cognitive-behavioral treatment as prerequisite to TFP. Patients who develop coping skills and techniques of stress management in such therapies may achieve enough stability to make participation in TFP possible.

"CRAVING" DISORDERS

For some borderline patients, a particular behavior, such as drinking, abusing drugs, overeating, starving, self-mutilation, spending money, or risky sexual behavior, provides such a ready solution for painful feelings that psychotherapeutic examination of such feelings is practically impossible. Some addictive behaviors compromise cognitive functioning to such an extent that exploratory psychotherapy is useless. In some such cases, the initial (contract-setting) phase of TFP may succeed in mobilizing the patient's willingness to use the treatment to bring these behaviors under control, or else to institute whatever adjunctive measures may be required to enable psychotherapy to proceed. A life-threatening anorexia, for instance, must be treated to the point of establishing a minimal normal weight before TFP can be undertaken. The anorectic patient must be told that TFP is a challenging procedure, that she must be in good physical condition to undertake it, and that it is a waste of time and effort to attempt treatment when her capacity to think clearly remains impaired by the metabolic imbalance produced by starvation. Once treatment has started, the anorectic patient is expected to maintain ongoing cooperation with the internist, and it is understood that if her weight falls below a safe level, therapy will be interrupted and appropriate treatment instituted until she regains a healthy weight.

The patient addicted to drugs or alcohol will require detoxification and a period of several months' sobriety, with an agreement to participate in Alcoholics Anonymous or some other appropriate support group, before TFP can begin. Ongoing involvement in a support group is usually required throughout the therapy in this group of patients. The treatment contract includes an agreement that the therapist and the internist will be in open communication at all times, that random urine screens will be part of ongoing treatment for substance abusers, and that therapy will be interrupted in the event of recurrence of substance abuse until sobriety has been reestablished. These patients thus require not only a preparatory treatment but also ongoing cotreatment with the internist during transference-focused psychotherapy.

Addictive behaviors that jeopardize a patient's financial solvency (such as gambling or excessive extravagance) can bring treatment to a halt if not brought under control by vigorous interpretive work early in the treatment process. If this contingency is foreseen during the assessment process, plans can be made for a preliminary phase of cognitive-behavioral treatment and possibly financial counseling before TFP begins.

Other forms of craving behavior may be less immediately threatening to the viability of the treatment and the well-being of the patient. They include overeating and obesity, shopping as a means of relieving anxiety, self-mutilation, unprotected promiscuity, and various other risk-taking behaviors such as smoking and irresponsibility with medications. Those behaviors that could endanger the patient or the course of treatment can usually be incorporated into the treatment contract and then are dealt with as transference enactments. Dangerously self-mutilating patients, for example, require a treatment contract that includes preventive visits to the emergency room when urges to injure the self are intolerable. TFP with such patients is made contingent on their willingness to be examined by a physician in the event of self-injury and to resume therapy only after the physician has ascertained that they are out of danger. Less threatening craving behaviors are treated as acting-out behaviors and are clarified, confronted, and dealt with interpretively.

INABILITY TO SUSTAIN MINIMAL FUNCTIONING BETWEEN SESSIONS

A patient's inability to sustain an image of the therapist or to remember what went on in the session may give rise to such intolerable anxiety that TFP cannot go on. Patients with this degree of difficulty are often treated in supportive psychotherapy with frequent sessions or sessions on demand. The usual outcome is the patient's escalating feelings of need and the therapist's exhaustion. A solution to the problem of sustaining functioning between sessions is the addition of a day hospital experience to the transference-focused therapy. This arrangement, like that of increasing the frequency of sessions, has the potential disadvantage of encouraging full-time patienthood as an alternative to normal life. The effectiveness of such a solution depends on maintaining clear goals for both concurrent treatment modalities, along with full communication between clinicians.

Some patients who cannot sustain functioning between sessions may need a course of treatment specifically designed to strengthen their coping skills (dialectic-behavior therapy, for example, to be described later in the chapter) as a prelude to TFP. Patients whose life situation is so chaotic and whose external supports are so meager that even a modicum of self-reflection is impossible require preliminary social work to secure the required supports before TFP can get under way.

DEPENDENCY, PARASITISM, AND "ENTITLEMENT"

Many borderline patients are prone to a degree of dependency that can be a formidable obstacle to progress in the treatment. Patients who have never held a job or have abandoned work in favor of dependence on their families or social agencies can adopt the position that "working" in therapy is all that is required of them in the pursuit of health. When challenged by the prospect of looking for work, these patients may drop out of treatment, experience intensification of suicidal or self-mutilating urges, or manifest alarming physical symptoms that can be difficult to diagnose.

For example, a patient who had failed to respond to years of supportive psychotherapy and who had used an eighteen-month period in a special hospital unit for treatment of borderline pathology as a theater for enactment of a fantasy of being "notoriously ill," told her new transference-focused therapist that she had been "thirsting for the session. I don't see how I can make it to the next session unless I can call you up and hear your voice." Thus, she attempted to lay the groundwork for another experience of "being in therapy" as an alternative to being in the world. It was essential for this patient to keep sessions at twice a week and to make regular employment a condition for continued treatment.

Another patient, who had been hospitalized after becoming depressed on being unable to tolerate the first week of a job in a nursing home, was considered ready for discharge after several months. The social worker helped her find a job as a night receptionist in a motel a ten-minute walk from the therapist's office, with a motel room as part of her salary. A few days before she was to be discharged, she developed vomiting and diarrhea that appeared to be disabling. The distraught therapist (who had gone to considerable trouble working with the social worker to arrange what seemed an ideal discharge plan) called the vocational rehabilitation counselor to report on the discouraging developments. "Never mind," he said, "we see this all the time. Just insist she go along with the plan." The patient moved into her new quarters, went to work, and recovered from the intestinal upset within twenty-four hours.

Regular work serves as a valuable balance to the preoccupation with psychotherapy, which can come to be seen by the patient as a substitute for normal living. Work constitutes a practice field for insights gained in therapy, provides material for the analysis of object relations in the sessions, serves as a testing ground for the progress made in the treatment, and eventually permits the patient to take financial responsibility for the therapy and to feel pride in so doing. In some cases, holding a full-time job or attending school full-time must be made a prerequisite for beginning TFP. In other cases, work becomes an early focus of the therapy; as the meanings of work become clarified through interpretation, the patient is able to sustain appropriate employment.

For example, a highly intelligent and capable woman took a succession of jobs during treatment, each time becoming ill or experiencing bosses and coworkers as malignant and the tasks as insuperably difficult. One job failure followed another until it became clear that, for this patient, who had been severely abused sexually and physically in her childhood, moving from the position of passive, cared-for (if humiliated) child to self-supporting adult meant identifying herself with the aggressor. To be an adult meant to be like the abusive parents, which stirred intense feelings of self-hatred and initiated a downward spiral of suicidal wishes, emergency room visits, absenteeism, and termination of employment.

It is not always possible to assess the seriousness of a patient's dependency or the steadfastness of her intent to make therapy a way of life without a trial of TFP. Some patients develop an interest in the treatment and an attachment to the therapist in the early phase of treatment sufficient to fuel a willingness to take seriously the therapist's insistence on work as an essential aspect of the therapeutic process. If not, working may have to be made a condition for continuing the treatment. The process of examining these issues and developing plans with the patient in advance for protecting the efficacy of the treatment may in itself constitute a preparatory brief psychotherapy that enables TFP to proceed.

MASOCHISM, ALEXITHYMIA, AND INABILITY TO TOLERATE ANXIETY

A group of patients with borderline pathology and pathological narcissism present with a frankly masochistic transference. Such patients often experience themselves as hurt and denigrated by the therapist in the initial interview and never return. Often the product of severe physical and psychological abuse, they may lack the intellectual vigor to differ openly with the therapist or the assertiveness to question or contest the treatment contract verbally. Their readiness to feel mistreated leaves them prone to massive misinterpretations of the therapist's utterances, which they cannot subject to open examination. Thus, they tend to drop out of treatment feeling wounded and unjustly treated. If they manage to remain in TFP for more than a few sessions, they tend to respond to interpretations as assaults, with upsurges of resentment that they cannot tolerate, reacting with massive denial and projection of their rage onto the therapist, who is now seen as a victimizer. In some patients, rage triggers dissociation as a means of warding off reactivation of intolerable memories of abuse. The result is that they cannot remember the session, and they enact their rage between sessions in impulsively destructive or self-destructive ways that can reach dangerous proportions. They either implicitly or explicitly blame the therapist for making them worse.

They often can be described as "alexithymic"—having an extremely limited repertoire of descriptors for their emotional states. They may, for example, use the term "upset" to mean any unpleasant emotional response, or they may describe themselves as "bad" when beginning to feel almost any emotion. Their access to memories and fantasies seems restricted to stereotyped, cartoonlike images and anecdotes, and their capacity for symbolic thinking and for making use of interpretations is minimal. The lack of nuance and richness in the inner life of these patients reflects the extremity of their need to maintain a split between hateful and benign internalized object representations. It may include specific difficulty in calling the image of the therapist to mind between sessions and remembering statements of the therapist that might have seemed useful during the session.

With their severely limited capacity to tolerate affects, poor impulse control, brittle defenses, and lack of verbal means of managing conflict, these patients are further compromised by the damaging effect of their masochistic stance on their interpersonal relationships. Their tendency to experience others as exploitive, unjust, and degrading deprives them of the social supports that might otherwise sustain them during the stresses inevitable in an interpretive treatment.

These patients typically present themselves as in desperate need of help but find the "help" represented by two psychotherapy sessions a week utterly insufficient. They describe and experience themselves as unsafe except when under the personal protection of the therapist, and they carry out a variety of self-destructive behaviors between sessions in the service either of relieving what they experience as intolerable anxiety or of extorting extra concern and attention from the therapist, or both.

A solution to the problem associated with the difficulties these patients have in sustaining even a minimally safe level of functioning between sessions has often been to shorten the interval between the sessions: patients have reported that in previous (failed) therapies they were provided with daily sessions—and sometimes even more than that—and had unlimited telephone access to the therapist. Such a solution usually makes matters worse instead of better. The more frequent sessions endorse a fantasy of barely being able to exist from one session to the next, with a consequent increasing constriction of the patient's life and a withering of capacities for work, creative and social activities, and life experience in general. Indeed, the tendency among borderline patients in general to substitute therapy for life is so powerful that spacing the sessions two or three days apart seems to be almost mandatory as a means of allowing room for consolidation of the effects of sessions and the integration of these effects into the patient's functioning in the world of work and social relationships.

INABILITY TO CONTAIN DANGEROUS BEHAVIOR

If the assessment process reveals imminently lethal or criminal behavior, TFP in an outpatient setting is contraindicated and hospitalization is a necessary preparatory treatment.

DERAILING TREATMENT WITH PSEUDO-EMERGENCIES

Patients with a history of coercing clinicians and family members to take care of them by creating crises may respond to the process of assessment and contract setting by becoming willing to enter a trial of TFP with the understanding that a "crisis" will result in whatever steps are necessary to deal with it, followed by referral for alternative treatment. The family must be involved in discussing this plan so as to be prepared for the possibility that the treatment may end quickly. The ongoing support of the family, with education about how to deal effectively with the patient's coercive behavior, may be effective. Unfortunately, many families have come to participate in the pattern of pseudo-emergencies and find it very difficult to alter their habitual response to the patient's alarming behaviors.

PREPARATORY TREATMENTS

For some patients, no formal preparatory treatment is necessary: assessment and contract setting suffice to introduce the patient to TFP and establish an adequate working relationship between patient and therapist. Generally speaking, the patients who can embark on TFP without preparatory treatment are intelligent and chronically and openly hostile people whose psychopathology includes a large admixture of pathological narcissism and who protest vigorously and contemptuously against the strictures of the initial treatment contract, denigrate the therapist unstintingly, threaten to end the treatment repeatedly, and in the early stages often engage defiantly in dangerous behavior between sessions. Yet they attend sessions regularly (often after some preliminary canceling that seems clearly in the service of testing the therapist's resolve when agreements about canceled sessions have formed part of the treatment contract) and rarely carry out their threats to end the treatment prematurely when these threats are skillfully handled. Although they may make urgent telephone calls to the therapist between sessions, these calls usually have the character of hostile intrusions on the therapist's privacy, or of attempts to control the therapist, rather than of expressions of panic or of inability to sustain an internal image of the therapist between sessions.

Such patients respond to the vigorous interpretation of their aggressive style of dealing with the therapist with a deepening of their interest in the treatment and a sometimes rapid, sometimes more gradual diminution of destructive behavior in their lives outside the sessions. Enactment of their negative transferences remains contained within the sessions until interpretive interventions have resolved them. Patients who are found during the assessment phase generally to fit this description characteristically respond well to TFP and require no preliminary or ancillary modalities of treatment.

THE ASSESSMENT PROCESS AS PREPARATORY TREATMENT

Most patients find a careful assessment of their problems and of the strengths they bring to the task of treatment to be a unique and extremely valuable experience. Such a process can be carried out by the prospective therapist, a separate diagnostician, or a diagnostic team and involves procedures that elucidate the severity of the symptoms, the history of the illness and of illness within the family, the nature of the patient's interpersonal relationships, the patient's sense of self, and his relationship to reality. The structural interview (Kernberg 1977) is one tool for accomplishing this assessment. Other approaches supplement diagnostic interviewing with a battery of self-administered tests and questionnaires and/or referral for standard psychological and neuropsychological testing. Because somatizing is such a frequent element in the defensive makeup of borderline patients, examination by an internist, employing whatever laboratory tests may be indicated, must always be part of the initial diagnostic study. By paying careful attention to all aspects of the patient's current psychosocial and physiological functioning, the clinician conveys a message that he is taking the patient and the problem very seriously, is not jumping to conclusions, and requires and expects the full and honest participation of the patient in a process of self-revelation and self-observation.

Even when the assessment requires only a few sessions (it may require more in complex cases), changes may occur similar to those seen in a brief psychotherapy. Patients may alter their attitude from one of cynical despair or pseudo-flippancy to a more earnest, hopeful, and committed position on treatment. Initial evasiveness, suspicion, and belligerence may give way to willingness to participate more openly. Or a patient who continues in a stance of contemptuous depreciation or oppositionalism nevertheless reveals serious involvement by showing up and carrying out required diagnostic procedures after having been desultory in previous treatments. When these kinds of changes occur in response to the assessment process, referral for TFP may be made directly if it is found to be indicated. Orientation to the treatment, of course, is part of this initial assessment: the treatment is described to the patient, who is implicitly assessing her own interest in it and her ability to participate. Discussion of the role of work and the rationale for making work a prerequisite for treatment is part of the preparatory phase.

CONTRACT SETTING AS PREPARATORY TREATMENT: CASE EXAMPLES

The development of the treatment contract constitutes another preparatory phase. As described elsewhere (Yeomans et al. 1992), the patient's way of responding to the setting up of a treatment contract is diagnostic and prognostic in itself. When a meaningful contract cannot be agreed on, the attempt to carry out TFP has to be abandoned in favor of some other modality, or none.

A patient who had participated seriously in the initial diagnostic study, understood the principles of TFP, and saw it as her only chance to overcome long-standing and disabling self-destructive behaviors concluded in her initial session with the clinician to whom she had been referred that he was the wrong therapist for her, that he was not kind, empathic, and flexible enough to be of help to her. On the grounds that such a hasty judgment probably reflected her fear of actually becoming involved in the treatment, and that she had been giving only lip service to its value, the therapist advised a trial period of several sessions before he would accede to her request for a new referral. The patient was furious and attempted to involve her family, her internist, and the original referring diagnostician in a campaign to be referred to another therapist. The struggle went on for several weeks but eventuated in the patient's reluctant agreement to a trial of treatment. In the sessions, her overt behavior continued to be contemptuous and rejecting, but she attended regularly and remained keenly engaged in the process of establishing the ground rules of the treatment. Her ability to participate in this initial phase of contract setting during the trial of therapy augured well for her eventual success in treatment.

Another patient who had resorted to severe but not lethal cutting of her genital area as a means of managing anxiety agreed to a plan whereby she would seek gynecological examination whenever she engaged in this behavior. Before the next session with the therapist could be scheduled, the gynecologist was to assure the therapist that no sutures were needed and no infection had resulted from the injury. The patient understood that this plan protected the psychotherapy, as the therapist would have difficulty maintaining objectivity if he was worried about her safety. Once having agreed to the plan, the patient stopped cutting herself, on the grounds that consulting the gynecologist about a self-inflicted injury would be too embarrassing.

COGNITIVE-BEHAVIORAL THERAPY IN SEQUENCE WITH TFP

A preliminary treatment in a cognitive-behavioral modality may be of considerable help in preparing patients who are too compromised by anxiety or impulsiveness to engage in transference-focused psychotherapy. As an example, the dialectic-behavior therapy (DBT) described by Marcia Linehan (1993) offers abundant support in the context of a highly structured program that combines didactic lectures, group sessions, and individual coaching with systematic written homework. Patients are taught to be aware of the fundamental instability of their thinking, emotional responses, and interpersonal behavior and to develop specific coping mechanisms to deal with this instability. An emphasis on overcoming their tendency to have judgmental responses to their own thoughts and feelings, as well as to others' behavior, can be useful in helping these patients tolerate the interpretations that will then be useful to them in TFP. Habits of self-observation (taught partly by means of strict recording of daily experiences of painful emotional states and self-damaging behavior) stand these patients in good stead in TFP: they are given detailed coaching in observing their inner states and overt responses and describing them both orally and in writing. For alexithymic patients, the development of verbal skills of this sort can be quite helpful.

In DBT, patients are systematically taught the concept of "treatment-interfering behavior," such as overeating—which prevents experiences of anxiety, thus making those experiences inaccessible to therapy—and importunate telephone calls that can erode a therapist's motivation to help the patient. Overspending that leads to self-impoverishment is another treatment-interfering behavior that patients are required to identify, observe, and cooperate with the therapist in bringing under control.

The DBT therapist tends to be informal and self-revelatory as compared to the psychoanalytically trained therapist. For example, a DBT therapist initiates telephone calls to patients from time to time as a means of expressing concern or demonstrating interest during periods when a patient is doing well (and hence may be fearing loss of entitlement to the therapist's involvement). No restrictions are placed on patients' access by telephone to the therapist unless it becomes clear that the patient's use of the telephone is impairing the therapist's capacity to remain appropriately involved in the treatment.

Many patients find the coping skills taught in DBT to be useful, although there are some patients who are capable of making unsuccessful and interminable cognitive-behavioral therapy a way of life. A patient who is unable to learn the coping skills taught in DBT or who chooses not to use them is probably a poor candidate for TFP, or indeed for therapy in general, although there is the occasional malignant narcissist who scornfully rejects the daily demands of DBT as drudgery but rises to the intellectual challenge she perceives in TFP.

Analytically Oriented Supportive Psychotherapy in Sequence with TFP: Case Examples

Borderline patients with mood disorders, ADD, PTSD, or dissociative disorders often require a period of supportive psychotherapy and medication trials before being able to benefit from TFP. Such an experience can foster the development of confidence in a cooperative enterprise with an expert clinician and can demonstrate to the patient the limits of what can be expected in the way of symptom relief from appropriate medication. Psychotherapy is supportive to borderline patients when it includes frank acknowledgment of the nature of their difficulty, solid information about what is known about causes and treatments, attention to the medical aspects of the patient's condition, and education about how to maintain health, including specific instructions about diet and exercise. In supportive therapy, the borderline patient is actively encouraged to maintain employment or persist in studies.

The psychoanalytically supportive therapist is aware of the patient's transference reactions and works to enable the patient to find socially acceptable channels for the discharge of aggression and safe ways of meeting needs for libidinal satisfaction in life outside therapy. Patients who function successfully in their work and are not overwhelmed by painful affects often respond favorably to supportive therapy.

A young executive sought treatment for sexual anesthesia. Indeed, it emerged that her entire body was unable to register touch: "If I touch my own arm, I can't feel it," she reported. She focused on her chief complaint in every session during the entire therapy, once a week for several years, never mentioning feelings for or fantasies about the therapist. She earnestly sought sexual experiences in the hope that with practice her symptoms would improve, and she reported on her experiments in detail and without affect. She spontaneously produced memories of sexual play in childhood with her brother and a period of being terrorized by a neighbor for a summer in preadolescence. She complained of her joyless life. The therapist recommended a practitioner of the Alexander technique as a possible avenue to recapturing body awareness. Soon after several such sessions, she informed the therapist that she had been aware of the pleasant feel and smell of the fresh air for the first time in her life. Over the ensuing year, she met a young man whose sexual preferences almost exactly matched the rituals of her childhood play with her brother. They married, established a lively and warm sexual relationship, and enjoyed their children.

Referral to TFP from supportive therapy is appropriate when the patient shows the capacity to benefit from interpretive work, while symptoms persist, and supportive psychotherapy seems to have reached a plateau. When there have been some substantial gains, the referral can feel to the patient like a kind of promotion or vote of confidence on the part of the clinician. But because the relationship with the supportive psychotherapist is a crucial element in a patient's response, referral inevitably constitutes a loss. Even if (as sometimes happens) the therapist remains on the case as the medication and backup doctor during the course of TFP, referral can feel to the patient like a rejection and requires careful preparation.

At one time, transference-focused therapy was thought to be endangered by patients' prior experiences of DBT or psychoanalytically based supportive psychotherapy, in that patients accustomed to a warmly directive approach would be unwilling to give this up in favor of the interpretive approach of TFP. Experience has shown that clear explanations of the method and rationale of TFP are readily grasped by patients who have had previous treatment of whatever sort. It is natural for patients to attribute failure to improve to their own shortcomings, and borderline patients may be particularly prone to such self-blame. It can be a relief and a motivating experience to be encouraged to consider that the treatment method rather than their own intransigence may account at least in part for the impasse they have reached. It has been our experience that whatever desires and expectations a patient brings to therapy are subject to clarification and interpretation in the course of ongoing treatment.

One patient who had been subjected to an incestuous relationship in childhood and adolescence and who had developed an extremely passive lifestyle (she was totally dependent on welfare and other social supports) was eventually hospitalized because of chronic self-mutilation. In the hospital, her intelligence and her capacity for strong attachments to helping figures were recognized. She improved enough to be referred to treatment in a day hospital based on DBT principles. Here she became attached to her therapist and, on the strength of this attachment, was willing to attempt for the first time in her life to apply for a job. After some months, the therapist thought she had made as much progress as she was likely to make with DBT and discussed the possibility of changing the treatment to TFP. The patient agreed, albeit with considerable trepidation. In the early phase of the new treatment, she protested the strictness of the treatment contract, but she made steady progress and required no modification of TFP procedures.

TFP IN SEQUENCE
WITH PSYCHOANALYSIS

Sometimes transference-focused psychotherapy becomes a preparation for standard psychoanalysis. The indications for analysis may become clear in these cases as the borderline patient's capacity to endure anxiety and frustration is strengthened in TFP, the ability to confront inner conflicts increases, and the characteristically split self and object representations are integrated. As these objectives of TFP are met, a patient's creativity and intellectual strivings may be freed up, but their fulfillment may be prevented by neurotic conflicts. At the point at which TFP begins to resemble standard psychoanalysis, it is reasonable for the patient and therapist to consider termination with the possibility in mind of referral for analysis once the termination is accomplished.

SUPPORTIVE PSYCHOTHERAPY
IN SEQUENCE WITH TFP

When it becomes clear that TFP is ineffective or harmful to a patient who nevertheless suffers from borderline pathology, plans should be made for shifting to supportive treatment.

Patients who are limited intellectually and who think so concretely as to be unable to grasp the "as-ifness" of interpretations are unlikely to benefit from TFP and may be helped considerably by DBT or supportive therapy.

Some patients who are unwilling or unable to commit themselves to the regular sessions and other aspects of the TFP treatment frame may be able to benefit from a supportive treatment on demand. For example, a young woman with severe identity diffusion and intense feelings of shame experienced excruciating distress in the face of the expectation that she would speak spontaneously in TFP. She could make contact with the therapist only by bringing up physical complaints and trying to elicit the therapist's medical opinion. She dropped out of treatment but called the therapist several years later to request, not "treatment," but "conversations." The therapist agreed, and they proceeded to meet regularly, talking in an open and informal way about her work, her boyfriend, and sometimes her inner life. The therapist freely expressed her opinions but refrained from offering transference interpretations. This phase of the treatment was noteworthy for the patient's increasing comfort and spontaneity and the increasing enjoyment of her daily life.

*   *   *

To summarize, transference-focused psychotherapy may be carried out successfully with some patients without a supportive preparatory treatment and without such concomitant support as Alcoholics Anonymous, day treatment, or monitoring by the internist. For other patients, considerable preparation is necessary, particularly if the illness includes addictive behaviors or eating disorders. Such cases require ongoing supervision by the internist and close collaboration between the internist and therapist. Finally, transference-focused psychotherapy may constitute a preparatory phase for psychoanalysis for patients who need and can benefit from a more intensive therapy when the goals of TFP have been achieved.

References

Ainsworth, M., M. C. Blehar, E. Waters, and S. Wall. 1978. *Patterns of Attachment: A Psychological Study of the Strange Situation.* Hillsdale, N.J.: Lawrence Erlbaum.

Akhtar, S. 1992. *Broken Structures: Severe Personality Disorders and Their Treatment.* Northvale, N.J.: Jason Aronson.

Akiskal, H. S. 1981. "Subaffective Disorders: Dysthymic, Cyclothymic, and Bipolar II Disorders in the 'Borderline' Realm." *Psychiatric Clinics of North America* 4, 25–46.

Altman, L. 1969. *The Dream in Psychoanalysis.* New York: International Universities Press.

American Psychiatric Association. 1994. *Diagnostic and Statistical Manual of Mental Disorders.* 4th ed. Washington, D.C.: American Psychiatric Association.

Appelbaum, A. H. 1996. "Why Traumatized Patients Relapse." *Bulletin of the Menninger Clinic* 60, 450–63.

Appelbaum, A., and D. Diamond. 1993. "The Impact of Gender on Transference and Countertransference." *Psychoanalytic Inquiry* 13(2), 145–52.

Beebe, B., and F. M. Lachmann. 1998. "Co-constructing Inner and Relational Processes: Self and Mutual Regulation in Infant Research and Adult Treatment." *Psychoanalytic Psychology* 15, 480–516.

Bergmann, M. S. 1994. "The Challenge of Erotized Transference to Psychoanalytic Technique." *Psychoanalytic Inquiry* 14(4), 499–519.

Bion, W. R. 1967. *Second Thoughts.* London: Heinemann.

———. 1968. "On Arrogance." In *Second Thoughts: Selected Papers on Psychoanalysis* (pp. 86–92). New York: Basic Books. (Originally published in 1957)

Bleuler, E. 1908. *Textbook of Psychiatry.* Translated by A. A. Brill. New York: Macmillan.

Blum, H. P. 1973. "The Concept of Erotized Transference." *Journal of the American Psychoanalytic Association* 29, 61–76.

Bowlby, J. 1969. *Attachment and Loss.* Vol. 1, *Attachment.* New York: Basic Books.

———. 1973. *Attachment and Loss.* Vol. 2, *Separation.* New York: Basic Books.

———. 1977. "The Making and Breaking of Affectional Bonds. I. Aetiology and Psychopathology in the Light of Attachment Theory." *British Journal of Psychiatry,* 130, 201–10.

———. 1979. *The Making and Breaking of Affectional Bonds.* London: Tavistock Publications.

———. 1980. *Attachment and Loss.* Vol. 3, *Loss, Sadness, and Depression.* New York: Basic Books.

———. 1988. *A Secure Base: Parent-Child Attachment and Healthy Human Development.* New York: Basic Books.

Clarkin, J., F. Yeomans, and O. F. Kernberg. 1999. *Psychotherapy for Borderline Patients.* New York: Guilford Press.

———. 1999. *Transference-Focused Psychodynamic Therapy for Borderline Personality Disorder Patients.* New York: John Wiley.

Cleckley, H. 1941. *The Mask of Sanity.* St. Louis: Mosby.

Cloninger, C. R., D. M. Svrakic, and T. R. Przybeck. 1993. "A Psychobiological Model of Temperament and Character." *Archives of General Psychiatry* 50, 975–90.

Coccaro, E. F., L. J. Siever, H. M. Klar, et al. 1989. "Serotinergic Studies in Patients with Affective and Personality Disorders." *Archives of General Psychiatry* 46, 587–99.

Coid, J., B. Allolio, and L. H. Rees. 1983. "Raised Plasma Metenkephalin in Patients Who Habitually Mutilate Themselves." *Lancet* 2 (8349, September 3), 545–46.

Cornelius, J. R., P. H. Soloff, J. M. Perel, and R. F. Ulrich. 1993. "Continuation Pharmacotherapy of Borderline Personality Disorder with Haloperidol and Phenelzine." *American Journal of Psychiatry* 150, 1843–48.

Cowdry, R. W., and D. L. Gardner. 1988. "Pharmacotherapy of Borderline Personality Disorder." *Archives of General Psychiatry* 45, 111–19.

Deutsch, H. 1942. "Some Forms of Emotional Disturbance and Their Relationship to Schizophrenia." *Psychoanalytic Quarterly* 11, 301–21.

Diamond, D., L. Bartocetti, K. Levy, J. Clarkin, and P. Foelsch. 1999. "Attachment and Personality Organization: Measures of Structure and Change in TFP Treatment." Paper presented at the thirtieth annual meeting of the Society for Psychotherapy Research, Braga, Portugal (June).

Diamond, D., J. Clarkin, H. Levine, K. Levy, P. Foelsch, and F. Yeomans. 1999. "Borderline Conditions and Attachment: A Preliminary Report." *Psychoanalytic Inquiry* 19, 831–84.

Dozier, M. 1990. "Attachment Organization and Treatment Use for Adults with Serious Psychopathological Disorders." *Development and Psychopathology* 2, 47–60.

Dozier, M., and C. Tyrrell. 1998. "The Role of Attachment in the Therapeutic Relationship." In *Attachment Theory and Close Relationships,* edited by J. A. Simpson and W. S. Rholes (pp. 221–48). New York: Guilford Press.

Edelman, G. M. 1992. *Bright Air, Brilliant Fire: On the Matter of Mind.* New York: Basic Books.

Erntz, A. 1924. "Über Träume von Schizophrenen." *International Zeitschrift für Psychoanalyse* 10, 292–95.

Fairbairn, W. R. D. 1940. "Schizoid Factors in the Personality." In *An Object Relations Theory of Personality* (pp. 3–27). New York: Basic Books.

Farber, B. A., R. A. Lippert, and D. B. Nevas. 1995. "The Therapist as Attachment Figure." *Psychotherapy* 32, 204–12.

Figureroa, E., and K. R. Silk. 1997. "Biological Implications of Childhood Sexual Abuse in Borderline Personality Disorder." *Journal of Personality Disorders* 11, 71–92.

Foelsch, P., and O. Kernberg. 1998. "Transference-Focused Psychotherapy for Borderline Personality Disorders." *In Session: Psychotherapy in Practice* 4, 67–90.

Fonagy, P. 1998a. "Moments of Change in Psychoanalytic Theory: Discussion of a New Theory of Psychic Change." *Infant Mental Health Journal* 19, 346–53.

———. 1998b. "An Attachment Theory Approach to the Treatment of the Difficult Patient." *Bulletin of the Menninger Clinic* 62, 147–68.

Fonagy, P., and A. M. Higgitt. 1989. "A Developmental Perspective on Borderline Personality Disorder." *Revue Internationale Psychopathologie* 1, 125–59.

Fonagy, P., T. Leigh, M. Steele, H. Steele, R. Kennedy, G. Mattoon, M. Target, and A. Gerber. 1996. "The Relation of Attachment Status, Psychiatric Classification, and Response to Psychotherapy." *Journal of Clinical and Consulting Psychology* 64, 22–31.

Fonagy, P., H. Steele, M. Steele, K. Leigh, R. Kennedy, G. Mattoon, and M. Target. 1995. "Attachment, the Reflective Self, and Borderline States: The Predictive Specificity of the Main Attachment Interview in Pathological Emotional Development." In *Attachment Theory: Social, Developmental, and Clinical Perspectives*, edited by S. Goldberg, R. Muir, and J. Kerr (pp. 233–78). Hillsdale, N.J.: Lawrence Erlbaum.

Fonagy, P., M. Steele, H. Steele, and M. Target. 1997. "Reflective-Functioning Manual: Version 4.1. For Application to the Adult Attachment Interviews." University College London. Unpublished paper.

Fraiberg, A. 1983. "Pathological Defenses in Infancy." *Psychoanalytic Quarterly* 60, 612–35.

Frances, A., and J. F. Clarkin. 1981. "No Treatment as the Prescription of Choice." *Archives of General Psychiatry* 38, 542–45.

Freud, S. 1899. *The Interpretation of Dreams.* In *Standard Edition*, vol. 2. London: Hogarth Press. [The actual date of publication was 1899; the publisher added 1900 to the frontispiece to extend the copyright by one year.]

———. 1912. *The Dynamics of Transference.* In *Standard Edition*, vol. 12. London: Hogarth Press.

———. 1915. *Observations on Transference Love.* In *Standard Edition*, vol. 12. London: Hogarth Press.

———. 1917. *Mourning and Melancholia.* In *Standard Edition*, vol. 14. London: Hogarth Press.

Fyer, M. R., A. J. Frances, T. Sullivan, S. W. Hurt, and J. Clarkin. 1988. "Suicide Attempts in Patients with Borderline Personality Disorder." *American Journal of Psychiatry* 145, 737–39.

Gabbard, G. O. 1994. "Love and Lust in Erotic Transference." *Journal of the American Psychoanalytic Association* 42(2), 385–403.

Gabbard, G. O., and E. Lester. 1995. *Boundaries and Boundary Violations in Psychoanalysis.* New York: Basic Books.

Gage, F. H., Coates, P. W., Palmer, T. D., Kuhn, H. G., Fisher, L. J., Suhonen, J. O., Peterson, D. A., Suhr, S. T., Ray, J. (1995). "Survival and Differentiation of Adult

Neuronal Progenitor Cells Transplanted to the Adult Brain." *Proceedings National Academy of Science USA* 92, 11879–83.

Galenson, E. 1986. "Some Thoughts About Infant Psychopathology and Aggressive Development." *International Review of Psychoanalysis* 13, 349–54.

Gardner, A. R., and A. J. Gardner. 1975. "Self-mutilation, Obsessionality, and Narcissism." *British Journal of Psychiatry* 127, 127–32.

Gardner, D. L., P. B. Lucas, and R. W. Cowdry. 1990. "CSF Metabolites in Borderline Personality Disorder and Normal Controls." *Biology of Psychiatry* 28, 247–54.

George, C., N. Kaplan, and M. Main. 1985. "The Berkeley Adult Attachment Interview." Department of Psychology, University of California at Berkeley. Unpublished paper.

Goldberg, S. C., S. C. Schultz, P. M. Schultz, et al. 1986. "Borderline and Schizotypal Personality Disorders Treated with Low-Dose Thiothixine Versus Placebo." *Archives of General Psychiatry* 43, 680–86.

Goldsmith, H. H., I. I. Gottesman, and K. S. Lemery. 1997. "Epigenetic Approaches to Developmental Psychopathology." *Developmental Psychopathology* 9, 365–87.

Gudzer, J., J. Paris, P. Zelkowitz, and K. Marchessault. 1991. "Risk Factors for Borderline Pathology in Children." *Journal of the American Academy of Child and Adolescent Psychiatry* 35, 26–33.

Gunderson, J. 1990. "The Borderline Patient's Intolerance of Aloneness: Insecure Attachments and Therapist's Availability." *American Journal of Psychiatry* 153, 752–58.

Gunderson J. G., and G. R. Elliott. 1985. "The Interface Between Borderline Personality Disorder and Affective Disorder." *American Journal of Psychiatry* 142, 277–88.

Gunderson J. G., and K. A. Phillips. 1991. "A Current View of the Interface Between Borderline Personality Disorder and Depression." *American Journal of Psychiatry* 148, 967–75.

Hamilton, C. E. In press. "Continuity and Discontinuity of Attachment from Infancy Through Adolescence." *Child Development.*

Hare, R. D. 1993. "Without Conscience: The Disturbing World of the Psychopaths Among Us." New York: Pocket Books.

Hare, R. D., T. J. Harpur, A. R. Hakstian, S. D. Hart, and J. P. Newman. 1990. "The Revised Psychopathy Checklist: Reliability and Factor Structure." *Psychological Assessment* 2, 338–41.

Harlow, H., and M. K. Harlow. 1963. "A Study of Animal Affection." In *Primate Social Behavior,* edited by C. H. Southwick (pp. 174–84). Princeton, N.J.: Van Nostrand Rheinholdt.

Hazen, C., and P. R. Shaver. 1994. "Attachment as an Organizational Framework for Research on Close Relationships." *Psychological Inquiry* 5, 1–22.

Henderson, D. K. 1939. *Psychopathic States.* London: Chapman & Hall.

Henderson, D. K., and R. D. Gillespie. 1969. *Textbook of Psychiatry: For Students and Practitioners.* 10th ed. Revised by I. R. C. Batchelor. London: Oxford University Press.

Herman, J. L. 1993. "Sequelae of Prolonged and Repeated Trauma: Evidence for a Complex Post-traumatic Stress Syndrome (DESNOS)." In *Post-traumatic Stress Dis-*

order, DSM-IV and Beyond, edited by J. R. T. Davidson and E. Foa. Washington, D.C.: American Psychiatric Press.

Herman, J. L., J. C. Perry, and B. A. van der Kolk. 1989. "Childhood Trauma in Borderline Personality Disorder." *American Journal of Psychiatry* 146, 490–95.

Hesse, E. 1999. "The Adult Attachment Interview." In *Handbook of Attachment: Theory, Research, and Clinical Applications,* edited by J. Cassidy and P. R. Shaver (pp. 395–433). New York: Guilford Press.

Hesse, E., and M. Main. 1999. "Second-Generation Effects of Unresolved Trauma in Nonmaltreating Parents: Dissociated, Frightened, and Threatening Parental Behavior." *Psychoanalytic Inquiry* 19(5), 481–541.

Hill, D. 1994. "The Special Place of the Erotic Transference in Psychoanalysis." *Psychoanalytic Inquiry* 14(4), 483–99.

Holmes, J. 1995. "Something There Is That Doesn't Love a Wall: John Bowlby, Attachment Theory, and Psychoanalysis." In *Attachment Theory: Social, Developmental, and Clinical Perspectives,* edited by S. Goldberg, R. Muir, and J. Kerr (pp. 19–43). Hillsdale, N.J.: Analytic Press.

———. 1996. *Attachment, Intimacy, and Autonomy: Using Attachment Theory in Adult Psychotherapy.* Northvale, N.J.: Jason Aronson.

———. 1997. "Too Early, Too Late: Endings in Psychotherapy—An Attachment Perspective." *British Journal of Psychotherapy* 14, 159–71.

———. 1998. "The Changing Aims of Psychoanalytic Psychotherapy." *International Journal of Psychoanalysis* 79, 227–40.

Jacobson, E. 1971. "Acting out the Urge to Betray in Paranoid Patients." In *Depression* (pp. 302–18). New York: International Universities Press.

———. 1991. *Depression: Comparative Studies of Normal, Neurotic, and Psychotic Conditions.* New York: International Universities Press.

Kavoussi, R. J., J. Liu, and E. F. Coccaro. 1994. "An Open Trial of Sertraline in Personality Disordered Patients with Impulsive Aggression." *Journal of Clinical Psychiatry* 55, 137–41.

Kemperman, I., M. J. Russ, and E. Shearin. 1997. "Self-injurious Behavior and Mood Regulation in Borderline Patients." *Journal of Personality Disorders* 11, 146–57.

Kernberg, O. F. 1967. "Borderline Personality Organization." *Journal of the American Psychoanalysis Association* 15, 641–85.

———. 1975. *Borderline Conditions and Pathological Narcissism.* New York: Jason Aronson.

———. 1976. *Object Relations Theory and Clinical Psychoanalysis.* London. Jason Aronson.

———. 1977. "The Structural Diagnosis of Borderline Personality Organization." In *Borderline Personality Disorders: The Concept, the Syndrome, the Patient,* edited by P. Hartocollis. New York: International Universities Press.

———. 1980. *Internal World and External Reality.* New York: Jason Aronson.

———. 1984. *Severe Personality Disorders: Psychotherapeutic Strategies.* New Haven, Conn.: Yale University Press.

———. 1992. *Aggression in Personality Disorders and Perversions*. New Haven, Conn.: Yale University Press.

———. 1994a. "Aggression Trauma and Hatred in the Treatment of Borderline Patients." *Psychiatric Clinics of North America* 17, 701–14.

———. 1998. *Ideology, Conflict, and Leadership in Groups and Organizations*. New Haven, Conn.: Yale University Press.

———. 1999. "The Influence of the Gender of Patient and Analyst in the Psychoanalytic Situation." Unpublished paper.

Kernberg, O. F., M. Selzer, H. W. Koenigsberg, A. Carr, and A. Appelbaum. 1989. *Psychodynamic Psychotherapy for Borderline Patients*. New York: Basic Books.

Kjelsberg, E., P. H. Eikeseth, and A. A. Dahl. 1991. "Suicide in Borderline Patients: Predictive Factors." *Acta Psychiatra Scandinavia* 84, 283–87.

Klein, M. 1946. "Notes on Some Schizoid Mechanisms." In *Envy and Gratitude and Other Works, 1946–1963* (pp. 1–24). New York: Free Press.

———. 1957. *Envy and Gratitude*. New York: Basic Books.

Kobak, R., and P. R. Shaver. 1987. "Strategies for Maintaining Felt Security: Implications for Adaptation and Psychopathology." Paper prepared for the Conference on Attachment and Loss in Honor of John Bowlby's Eightieth Birthday, London (June).

Koenigsberg, H. W. 1993. "Combining Psychotherapy and Pharmacotherapy in the Treatment of Borderline Patients." In *American Psychiatric Press Review of Psychiatry*, edited by J. M. Oldham, M. B. Riba, and A. Tasman (vol. 12, pp. 541–63). Washington, D.C.: American Psychiatric Press.

———. 1997. "Integrating Psychotherapy and Pharmacotherapy in the Treatment of Borderline Personality Disorder." *In Session: Psychotherapy in Practice* 3, 39–56.

Koenigsberg, H. W., I. Anwunah, A. S. New, V. Mitropoulou, F. Schopick, and L. J. Siever. 1999. "Relationship Between Depression and Borderline Personality Disorder." *Depression and Anxiety* 10, 158–67.

Kohut, H. 1971. *The Analysis of the Self*. New York: International Universities Press.

Kolb, L. C. 1987. "Neurophysiological Hypothesis Explaining Post-Traumatic Stress Disorder." *American Journal of Psychiatry* 144, 988–95.

Kretschmer, E. 1925. *Physique and Character*. Translated by W. J. H. Sprott. New York: Harcourt Brace.

Kroll, J. 1993. *PTSD/Borderlines in Therapy: Finding the Balance*. New York: W. W. Norton.

Lichtenberg, J. 1999. "Discussion." *Psychoanalytic Inquiry* 19, 4, 647–661.

Liebowitz, M. R., and D. F. Klein. 1981. "Interrelationship of Hysteroid Dysphoria and Borderline Personality Disorder." *Psychiatric Clinics of North America* 4, 67–87.

Linehan, M. M. 1993. *Cognitive-Behavioral Treatment of Borderline Personality Disorder*, edited by A. Frances. New York: Guilford Press.

Links, P. S., M. Steiner, I. Boiago, and D. Irwin. 1990. "Lithium Therapy for Borderline Patients: Preliminary Findings." *Journal of Personality Disorders* 4, 173–81.

Liotti, G. 1995. "Disorganized/Disoriented Attachment in the Psychotherapy of the Dissociative Disorders." In *Attachment Theory: Social, Developmental, and Clinical*

Perspectives, edited by S. Goldberg, R. Muir, and J. Kerr (pp. 343–67). Hillsdale, N.J.: Analytic Press.

———. 1999. "Understanding the Dissociative Processes: The Contributions of Attachment Theory." *Psychoanalytic Inquiry* 19(5) 757–783.

Lyons-Ruth, K. 1999. "The Two-Person Unconscious: Intersubjective Dialogue, Enactive Relational Representation, and the Emergence of New Forms of Relational Organization." *Psychoanalytic Inquiry* 19(4), 576–617.

Mackie, A. J. 1981. "Attachment Theory: Its Relevance to the Therapeutic Alliance." *British Journal of Medical Psychology* 54, 201–12.

Main, M. 1991. "Metacognitive Knowledge, Metacognitive Monitoring, and Singular (Coherent) Versus Multiple (Incoherent) Models of Attachment: Findings and Directions for Future Research." In *Attachment Across the Life Cycle,* edited by C. M. Parkes, J. Stevenson-Hinde, and P. Marris (pp. 127–59). London: Routledge.

———. 1995. "Recent Studies in Attachment: Overview with Selected Implications for Clinical Work." In *Attachment Theory: Social, Development, and Clinical Perspectives,* edited by S. Goldberg, R. Muir, and J. Kerr (pp. 407–475). Hillsdale, N.J.: Lawrence Erlbaum.

———. 1999. "Epilogue: Attachment Theory: Eighteen Points with Suggestions for Future Studies." In *Handbook of Attachment: Theory, Research, and Clinical Applications,* edited by J. Cassidy and P. R. Shaver (pp. 885–887). New York: Guilford Press.

Main, M., and R. Goldwyn. 1998. "Adult Attachment Scoring and Classifications System" (scoring manual). University of California at Berkeley, Department of Psychology. Unpublished paper.

Main, M., and E. Hesse. 1990. "Parents' Unresolved Traumatic Experiences Are Related to Infant Disorganized Attachment Status: Is Frightened and/or Frightening Parental Behavior the Linking Mechanism?" In *Attachment in the Preschool Years: Theory, Research, and Intervention,* edited by M. T. Greenberg, D. Cicchetti, and E. M. Cummings (pp. 161–82). Chicago: University of Chicago Press.

Main, M., N. Kaplan, and J. Cassidy. 1985. "Security in Infancy, Childhood, and Adulthood: A Move to the Level of Representation." In *Growing Points in Attachment Theory and Research,* edited by I. Bretherton and E. Waters (pp. 66–104). Monograph for the Society for Research in Child Development. Chicago: University of Chicago Press.

Main, M., and H. Morgan. 1996. "Disorganization and Disorientation in Infant Strange Situation Behavior: Phenotypic Resemblance to Dissociative States." In *Handbook of Dissociation: Theoretical, Empirical, and Clinical Perspectives,* edited by L. K. Michelson and W. J. Ray (pp. 107–37). New York: Plenum Press.

Main, M., and D. Weston. 1981. "The Quality of the Toddler's Relationship to Mother and to Father Related to Conflict Behavior and the Readiness to Establish New Relationships." *Child Development* 52, 932–40.

Maltsberger, J. T., and D. H. Buie. 1974. "Countertransference Hate in the Treatment of Suicidal Patients." *Archives of General Psychiatry* 30, 625–33.

Mann, J. J., and S. Kapur. 1991. "The Emergence of Suicidal Ideation and Behavior During Antidepressant Pharmacotherapy." *Archives of General Psychiatry* 48, 1027–33.

McEwen, B. S. 1994. "Corticosteroids and Hippocampal Plasticity." *Annals of the New York Academy of Science* 746, 134–42.

McEwen, B. S., E. A. Gould, and R. R. Sakai. 1992. "The Vulnerability of the Hippocampus to Protective and Destructive Effects of Glucocorticoids in Relation to Stress." *British Journal of Psychiatry* 16, 18–24.

Milgram, S. 1963. "Behavioral Study of Obedience." *Journal of Abnormal and Social Psychology* 67, 371–78.

Montgomery, S. A. 1987. "The Psychopharmacology of Borderline Personality Disorders." *Acta Psychiatra Belgium* 87, 260–66.

Norden, M. J. 1989. "Fluoxetine in Borderline Personality Disorder." *Progress in Neuropsychopharmacology and Biological Psychiatry* 13, 885–93.

Osofsky, J. D. 1988. "Affective Exchanges Between High-Risk Mothers and Infants." *International Journal of Psychoanalysis* 69, 221–32.

Parens, H. 1979. *The Development of Aggression in Early Childhood*. New York: Jason Aronson.

Paris, J. 1993. "Management of Acute and Chronic Suicidality in Patients with Borderline Personality Disorder." In *Borderline Personality Disorder: Etiology and Treatment,* edited by Joel Paris (pp. 373–83). Washington, D.C.: American Psychiatric Press.

———. 1994. *Borderline Personality Disorder: A Multidimensional Approach*. Washington, D.C.: American Psychiatric Press.

Paris, J., R. Brown, and D. Nowlis. 1989. "Predictors of Suicide in Borderline Personality Disorder." *Canadian Journal of Psychiatry* 34, 8–9.

Perry, J. C., and J. L. Herman. 1993. "Trauma and Defense in the Etiology of Borderline Personality Disorder." In Paris, J.(ed.), *Borderline Personality Disorders,* edited by Joel Paris (pp. 123–41). Washington, D.C.: American Psychiatric Press.

Perry, J. C., E. Banon, and F. Ianni. 1999. "Effectiveness of Psychotherapy for Personality Disorders." *American Journal of Psychiatry* 156, 1312–21.

Pinto, O. C., and H. S. Akiskal. 1998. "Lamotrigine as a Promising Approach to Borderline Personality: An Open Case Series Without Concurrent *DSM-IV* Major Mood Disorder." *Journal of Affective Disorders* 5, 333–43.

Plotsky, P. M., Meany, M. J. (1993). "Early Postnatal Experience Alters Hypothalamic Corticotropin-Releasing Factor (CRF) mRNA, Median Eminence CRF Content and Stress-Induced Release in Adult Rats." *Brain Research Molecular Brain Research* 18: 195–200.

Pope, H. G., J. M. Jonas, J. I. Hudson, et al. 1983. "The Validity of *DSM-III* Borderline Personality Disorder: A Phenomenologic, Family History, Treatment Response, and Long-term Follow-up Study." *Archives of General Psychiatry* 40, 23–30.

Post, R. M., and S. R. B. Weiss. 1997. "Emergent Properties of Neural Systems: How Focal Molecular Neurobiological Alteration Can Affect Behavior." *Developmental Psychopathology* 9, 907–29.

Putnam, F. W., and P. K. Trickett. 1997. "Psychobiological Effects of Sexual Abuse: A Longitudinal Study." *Annals of the New York Academy of Sciences* 821, 150–59.

Racker, H. 1968. *Transference and Countertransference.* London: Maresfield Library; New York: International Universities Press.

Resnick, P. J. 1998. "Malingering of Post-Traumatic Psychiatric Disorders." *Journal of Practical Psychiatry and Behavioral Health* 4, 329–39.

Richardson, G. A., and R. A. Moore. 1963. "On the Manifest Dream in Schizophrenia." *Journal of the American Psychoanalysis Association* 11, 281–302.

Rockland, L. H. 1992. *Supportive Psychotherapy for Borderline Patients: A Psychodynamic Approach.* New York: Guilford Press.

Rogers, J. H., T. A. Widiger, and A. Krupp. 1995. "Aspects of Depression Associated with Borderline Personality Disorder." *American Journal of Psychiatry* 152, 268–70.

Russell, D. E. 1989. *The Secret Trauma: Incest in the Lives of Girls and Women.* New York: Basic Books.

Rutter, M., J. Dunn, R. Plomin, E. Siminoff, A. Pickles, B. Maughan, J. Ormel, J. Meyer, and L. Eaves. 1997. "Integrating Nature and Nurture: Implications of Person-Environment Correlations for Developmental Psychopathology." *Developmental Psychopathology* 9, 335–64.

Sachsse, U. 1995. "The Psychodynamics of the Borderline Personality Disorder: An Outline." *Forum der Psychoanalyse: Zeitschrift Fuer Klinische Theroie und Praxis* 11(1), 50–61.

Salzman, C., A. N. Wolfson, A. Schatzberg, J. Looper, R. Henke, M. Albanese, J. Schwartz, and E. Miyawaki. 1995. "Effect of Fluoxetine on Anger in Symptomatic Volunteers with Borderline Personality Disorder." *Journal of Clinical Psychopharmacology* 15, 23–29.

Schlesinger, H. J. 1996. "The Fear of Being Left Half-cured." *Bulletin of the Menninger Clinic* 60, 428–49.

Schore, A. N. 1994. *Affect Regulation and the Origin of the Self.* Hillsdale, N.J.: Lawrence Erlbaum.

Selzer, M., H. W. Koenigsberg, and O. F. Kernberg. 1987. "The Initial Contract in the Treatment of Borderline Patients." *American Journal of Psychiatry* 144, 927–30.

Shengold, L. 1989. *Soul Murder: The Effects of Childhood Abuse and Deprivation.* New Haven, Conn.: Yale University Press.

Siever, L. 1993. "The Serotonin System and Aggressive Personality Disorder." *International Clinic of Psychopharmacology* 2 (November 8 supplement), 33–39.

Siever, L. J., and K. L. Davis. 1991. "A Psychobiological Perspective on Personality Disorders." *American Journal of Psychiatry* 148, 1647–58.

Siever, L. J., A. S. New, H. W. Koenigsberg, M. Buchsbaum, R. Yehuda, J. Gelernter, and R. Grossman. 1999. "The Psychobiology of Borderline Personality Disorder." Paper presented at the sixth annual meeting of the International Society for the Study of Personality Disorders, Geneva, Switzerland (September 17).

Siever, L. J., Buchsbaum, M. S., New, A. S., Speigel-Cohen, J., Wei, T., Hazlett, E. A., Sevin, E., Nunn, M., Mitropoulou, V. (1999a). "d,1-fenfluramine Response in

Impulsive Personality Disorder Assessed with [18F]flurodeoxyglucose Positron Emission Tomography." *Neuropsychopharmacology* 20: 413–423.

Silk, K. 1997. "Notes on the Biology of Borderline Personality Disorder." *Journal of the California Alliance for the Mentally Ill* 8, 15–17.

Silverman, J. M., L. Pinkham, T. B. Horvath, E. F. Coccaro, H. Klar, S. Schear, S. Apter, M. Davidson, R. C. Mohs, and L. J. Siever. 1991. "Affective and Impulsive Personality Disorder Traits in the Relatives of Patients with Borderline Personality Disorder." *American Journal of Psychiatry* 148, 1378–85.

Simeon, D., B. Stanley, A. Frances, J. J. Mann, R. Winchel, and M. Stanley. 1992. "Self-mutilation in Personality Disorders: Psychological and Biological Correlates." *American Journal of Psychiatry* 149, 221–26.

Slade, A. 1999. "Attachment Theory and Research: Implications for Theory and Practice of Individual Psychotherapy." In *Handbook of Attachment Theory and Research*, edited by J. Cassidy and P. Shaver (pp. 575–594). New York: Guilford Press.

Soloff, P. H. 1994. "Is There Any Drug Treatment of Choice for the Borderline Patient?" *Acta Psychiatra Scandinavia* 89(supplement 379), 50–55.

Soloff, P. H., G. Anselm, R. S. Nathan, et al. 1989. "Amitriptyline Versus Haloperidol in Borderlines: Final Outcomes and Predictors of Response." *Journal of Clinical Psychopharmacology* 9, 238–46.

Soloff, P. H., J. Cornelius, A. George, S. Nathan, J. M. Perel, and R. F. Ulrich. 1993. "Efficacy of Phenelzine and Haloperidol in Borderline Personality Disorder." *Archives of General Psychiatry* 50, 377–85.

Spitz, R. 1946. "Anaclitic Depression." *Psychoanalytic Study of the Child* 2, 313–42.

Stein, G. 1992. "Drug Treatment of Personality Disorders." *British Journal of Psychiatry* 161, 167–84.

Steinberg, B. J., R. Trestman, V. Mitropoulou, M. Serby, E. F. Coccaro, S. Weston, M. deVegvar, and L. J. Siever. 1997. "Depressive Response to Physostigmine Challenge in Borderline Personality Disorder Patients." *Neuropsychopharmacology* 17, 264–73.

Stern, D. 1999. "Personality and Emotional Development." Paper presented at the sixth annual meeting of the International Society for the Study of Personality Disorders, Geneva, Switzerland (September 17).

Stern, D. N., L. W. Sander, J. P. Nahum, A. M. Harrison, K. Lyons-Ruth, A. Morgan, N. Bruschweiler-Stern, and E. Z. Tronick. 1998. "Non-interpretive Mechanisms in Psychoanalytic Therapy: The 'Something More' Than Interpretation." *International Journal of Psychoanalysis* 79, 902–21.

Stone, M. H. 1977. "Factitious Illness: Psychological Findings and Treatment Recommendations." *Bulletin of the Menninger Clinic* 4, 239–54.

———. 1979. "Dreams of Fragmentation and of the Death of the Dreamer." *Psychopharmacology Bulletin* 15, 12–14.

———. 1980. *The Borderline Syndromes: Constitution, Personality, and Adaptation*. New York: McGraw-Hill.

———. 1983. "Abnormalities of Personality." *Journal of the American Academy of Psychoanalysis* 11, 87–111.

————. 1985. "Disturbances in Sex and Love in Borderline Patients." In *Sexuality: New Perspectives*, edited by Z. DeFries, R. C. Friedman, and R. Corn. Westport, Conn.: Greenwood Press.

————. 1990. *The Fate Of Borderline Patients*. New York: Guilford Press.

————. 1993a. "Paradoxes in the Management of Suicidality in Borderline Patients." *American Journal of Psychotherapy* 47, 255–72.

————. 1993b. "Etiology of Borderline Personality Disorder: Psychobiological Factors Contributing to an Underlying Irritability." In *Borderline Personality Disorders*, edited by J. Paris (pp. 87–101). Washington, D.C.: American Psychiatric Press.

Szajnberg, N. M., and P. M. Crittenden. 1997. "The Transference Refracted Through the Lens of Attachment." *Journal of the American Academy of Psychoanalysis* 25(3), 409–38.

Travin, S., and B. Protter. 1984. "Malingering and Malingering-like Behavior: Some Clinical and Conceptual Issues." *Psychiatric Quarterly* 56, 189–97.

Van der Kolk, B. A. 1987. *Psychological Trauma*. Washington, D.C.: American Psychiatric Press.

————. 1989. "Compulsion to Repeat the Trauma: Reenactment, Revictimization, and Masochism." *Psychiatric Clinics of North America* 12, 389–412.

Van der Kolk, B. A., and R. E. Fisler. 1994. "Childhood Abuse and Neglect and Loss of Self-regulation." *Bulletin of the Menninger Clinic* 58, 145–68.

Van der Kolk, B., A. C. McFarlane, and L. Weisaeth. 1996. *Traumatic Stress*. New York: Guilford Press.

Van IJzendoorn, M. H., and M. J. Bakermans-Kranenburg. 1995. "Attachment Representations in Mothers, Fathers, Adolescents, and Clinical Groups: A Meta-analytic Search for Normative Data." *Journal of Consulting and Clinical Psychology* 64, 8–21.

Waters, E., S. K. Merrick, D. Treboux, J. Crowell, and L. Albersheim. In press. "Attachment Security from Infancy to Early Adulthood: A Twenty-Year Longitudinal Study." *Child Development*.

Winnicott, D. W. 1960. "Ego Distortion in Terms of True and False." In *The Maturational Process and the Facilitating Environment* (pp. 140–52). New York: International Universities Press.

————. 1965. *The Maturation Processes and the Facilitating Environment*. New York. International Universities Press.

Wrye, H. K. 1993. "Erotic Terror: Male Patients' Horror of the Maternal Erotic Transference." *Psychoanalytic Inquiry* 13(2), 240–57.

Wrye, H. K., and J. K. Welles. 1989. "The Maternal Erotic Transference." *International Journal of Psychoanalysis* 70(4), 673–84.

Yeomans, F., J. Hull, and J. Clarkin. 1994. "Risk Factors for Self-damaging Acts in a Borderline Population." *Journal of Personality Disorders* 8, 10–16.

Yeomans, F. E., M. A. Selzer, and J. Clarkin. 1992. *Treating the Borderline Patient: A Contract-Based Approach*. New York: Basic Books.

Zanarini, M. C., F. R. Frankenburg, E. D. Dubo, A. E. Sickel, A. Trikha, A. Levin, and V. Reynolds. 1998. "Axis I Comorbidity of Personality Disorders." *American Journal of Psychiatry* 155, 1733–39.

Zetzel, E. 1968. "The So-called Good Hysteric." *International Journal of Psychoanalysis* 49, 256–60.

Zhang, L. X., G. Q. Xing, S. Levine, R. M. Post, and R. A. Smith. 1997. "Maternal Deprivation Induces Neuronal Death." *Society of Neuroscience Abstracts* 23, 1113.

Zinoviev, A. 1984. *The Reality of Communism.* New York: Schocken.

Index